# Methods of Pesticide Exposure Assessment

## NATO • Challenges of Modern Society

A series of edited volumes comprising multifaceted studies of contemporary problems facing our society, assembled in cooperation with NATO Committee on the Challenges of Modern Society.

---

Recent volumes in this series:

Volume 3 AIR POLLUTION MODELING AND ITS APPLICATION II
Edited by C. De Wispelaere

Volume 4 HAZARDOUS WASTE DISPOSAL
Edited by John P. Lehman

Volume 5 AIR POLLUTION MODELING AND ITS APPLICATION III
Edited by C. De Wispelaere

Volume 6 REMOTE SENSING FOR THE CONTROL OF MARINE POLLUTION
Edited by Jean-Marie Massin

Volume 7 AIR POLLUTION MODELING AND ITS APPLICATION IV
Edited by C. De Wispelaere

Volume 8 CONTAMINATED LAND: Reclamation and Treatment
Edited by Michael A. Smith

Volume 9 INTERREGIONAL AIR POLLUTION MODELING: The State of the Art
Edited by S. Zwerver and J. van Ham

Volume 10 AIR POLLUTION MODELING AND ITS APPLICATION V
Edited by C. De Wispelaere, Francis A. Schiermeier, and Noor V. Gillani

Volume 11 AIR POLLUTION MODELING AND ITS APPLICATION VI
Edited by Han van Dop

Volume 12 RISK MANAGEMENT OF CHEMICALS IN THE ENVIRONMENT
Edited by Hans M. Seip and Anders B. Heiberg

Volume 13 AIR POLLUTION MODELING AND ITS APPLICATION VII
Edited by Han van Dop

Volume 14 HEALTH AND MEDICAL ASPECTS OF DISASTER PREPAREDNESS
Edited by John C. Duffy

Volume 15 AIR POLLUTION MODELING AND ITS APPLICATION VIII
Edited by Han van Dop and Douw G. Steyn

Volume 16 DIOXIN PERSPECTIVES: A Pilot Study on International Information Exchange on Dioxins and Related Compounds
Edited by Erich W. Bretthauer, Heinrich W. Kraus, and Alessandro di Domenico

Volume 17 AIR POLLUTION MODELING AND ITS APPLICATION IX
Edited by Han van Dop and George Kallos

Volume 18 AIR POLLUTION MODELING AND ITS APPLICATION X
Edited by Sven-Erik Gryning and Millán M. Millán

Volume 19 METHODS OF PESTICIDE EXPOSURE ASSESSMENT
Edited by Patricia B. Curry, Sesh Iyengar, Pamela A. Maloney, and Marco Maroni

# Methods of Pesticide Exposure Assessment


**Edited by**

**Patricia B. Curry**
*Health Canada*
*Ottawa, Ontario, Canada*

**Sesh Iyengar**
*Zeneca Agro*
*Stoney Creek, Ontario, Canada*

**Pamela A. Maloney**
*Health Canada*
*Ottawa, Ontario, Canada*

**and**

**Marco Maroni**
*International Centre for Pesticide Safety*
*Busto Garolfo, Italy*



Published in cooperation with
NATO Committee on the Challenges of Modern Society

**PLENUM PRESS • NEW YORK AND LONDON**

Library of Congress Cataloging-in-Publication Data

Methods of pesticide exposure assessment / edited by Patricia B. Curry ... [et al.].
p. cm. -- (NATO challenges of modern society ; v. 19)
"Published in cooperation with NATO Committee on the Challenges of Modern Society".
"Proceedings of a Workshop on Methods of Pesticide Exposure Assessment, held Oct. 5-8, 1993, in Ottawa, Ontario, Canada" -- Copr. p.
Includes bibliographical references and index.
ISBN 0-306-45130-1
1. Pesticides--Toxicology--Congresses. 2. Health risk assessment--Congresses. I. Curry, P. B. II. Series.
RA1270.P4M476 1995
615.9'02--dc20 95-25134
CIP

Proceedings of a Workshop on Methods of Pesticide Exposure Assessment, held October 5–8, 1993, in Ottawa, Ontario, Canada

Developed from a Workshop sponsored by Health Canada and the North Atlantic Treaty Organisation and officially supported by the United States Environmental Protection Agency and the Organisation for Economic Cooperation and Development.

ISBN 0-306-45130-1


A Division of Plenum Publishing Corporation
233 Spring Street, New York, N. Y. 10013



Printed in the United States of America

# PREFACE

This book is a summary of the presentations and discussions at the Workshop on Methods of Pesticide Exposure Assessment held in Ottawa, Canada, on October 5-8, 1993. The event was a joint effort of Health Canada and the North Atlantic Treaty Organisation and was officially supported by the United States Environmental Agency and the Organisation for Economic Co-operation and Development (OECD). The goal of the workshop was to examine current issues in the field of pesticide exposure assessment with the aim of reaching an internationally harmonized approach to methods of exposure assessment.

With regulatory agencies of OECD Member countries moving towards the harmonization of data requirements, it was timely and beneficial to bring together international experts in the field of pesticide exposure assessment to discuss current issues. Approximately 60 delegates and 20 observers participated, including individuals from 15 different countries representing academia, government, industry and international organizations.

A guidance document on methods of pesticide exposure assessment was presented for critique and discussion as a means to achieving the goal of international harmonization. After extensive discussion, the workshop delegates agreed in principle to procedures for revising the guidance document. Following revision and further review by a designated peer review group, the revised document will be submitted to the OECD for consideration as a draft OECD Guidance Document on pesticide exposure assessment methods. Both the revised and original documents are included in these proceedings.

A tier approach to the use of exposure assessment in the risk assessment of pesticides was also presented and discussed. Field studies as outlined in the guidance document discussed above form one component of this approach. Another component of the tier approach is the use of surrogate exposure data. Two databases that may supply surrogate exposure data, the Pesticide Handlers Exposure Database and the predictive model being developed in the European Union (formerly the European Community), were compared.

The workshop concluded with discussion on future methods of exposure assessment. Several presentations were made on biomarkers of exposure and their usefulness in the field of pesticide exposure assessment, a new and exciting area in the field of exposure assessment.

This workshop created an opportunity to maintain dialogue amongst experts in the field of pesticide exposure assessment. A major outcome of the workshop was the agreement in principle by delegates from 15 countries to a procedure for the revision of the guidance document on pesticide exposure assessment methods for presentation as a proposed Guidance Document to the OECD. The workshop also resulted in two major recommendations.

1. The need for further work and discussion into the usefulness of biomarkers for determining worker exposure was identified.

2. The need for further discussion and perhaps an international meeting on the use of exposure assessment in risk assessment was agreed to.

P.B. Curry, S. Iyengar, P. Maloney, and M. Maroni

## ACKNOWLEDGEMENTS

Sincere thanks is extended to all those who helped make this workshop a success. The workshop chair was Deirdre Morison of Health Canada. The workshop organizing committee included D. Morison, S. Iyengar, P. Curry and P. Maloney of Health Canada; M. Maroni of the North Atlantic Treaty Organisation; A. Nielsen of the United States Environmental Protection Agency; J. van Hemmen of TNO Nutrition and Food Research Institute in The Netherlands and C. Maas of The Netherlands Ministry of Social Affairs and Employment. The efforts of the session leaders for chairing and guiding the discussion in their sessions and the rapporteurs for recording the discussion are gratefully acknowledged. The workshop coordinators, H. Lamadeleine, V. Nash-Moore and J. Lowe of Golden Planners Inc., were indispensable throughout the workshop as well as during the workshop planning stages. Finally, Lois Lemieux and Debbie Miller are thanked for diligent word processing and Plenum Press for their patience in awaiting the completion of these proceedings.

## CONTENTS

## SESSION TWO — PESTICIDE EXPOSURE DATABASES



## SESSION THREE — THE TIER APPROACH

## SESSION FOUR — BIOMARKERS OF EXPOSURE



## APPENDICES

# PESTICIDE EXPOSURE ASSESSMENT: PAST, PRESENT AND FUTURE

John P. Worgan and Sylvester Rozario

Health Canada
Chemical Evaluation Division
Rm 2702, Main Statistics Canada Bldg.
Tunney's Pasture
Ottawa, Ontario K1A 0L2
Canada

## INTRODUCTION

The purpose of this paper is to provide a brief overview of the past and present accomplishments and possible future directions of the field of pesticide exposure assessment. Furthermore, this paper is meant to provide the background and set the stage for discussion of the four main workshop goals, namely to:

i) review and revise a draft guidance document on pesticide exposure assessment methods,
ii) identify and discuss common principles between pesticide exposure databases/models that are available or being developed,
iii) examine the use of the tiered approach in the regulation of pesticides, and
iv) discuss the usefulness of biomarkers for estimating dose to individuals occupationally exposed to pesticides.

Pesticides are toxic, biologically active chemicals that are intentionally released into the environment to control pests such as weeds, insects and fungi. They are extensively used in agriculture to improve productivity and there has been a upward trend in use over the past four decades. In Canada there are presently 482 registered active ingredients formulated in 6,686 end-use products. Since the 1940's when synthetic organic pesticides were first introduced there has been a significant increase in pesticide sales and use. For example the number of acres treated with herbicides in Canada increased 250% to 53 million acres from 1970 to 1980. The number of farms using herbicides has increased from 40% in 1971 to 50% in 1991, though a drop from 59% in 1986 was observed[1]. Similar trends have been reported for the United States and other developed countries. In 1985, worldwide consumption of pesticides was estimated at about 3 million tonnes. The major applications of pesticides in the world in 1985 were herbicides (46%), insecticides (31%) and fungicides (18.4%)[2]. One can infer that this increase in pesticidal use over the years can result in increased exposure potential thus necessitating a full understanding of the risks associated with these products.

*Methods of Pesticide Exposure Assessment*, Edited by
P.B. Curry *et al.*, Plenum Press, New York, 1995

The risks of these products depend on their inherent toxicity and on the level of exposure. This is true not only for workers but also the general public, although the routes of uptake may differ. Determination of the health risk for applicators and other pesticide handlers requires an understanding of the toxicity of the pesticide and knowledge of the use pattern including route, duration and magnitude of exposure.

Exposure to pesticides can occur by three main routes, namely dermal, inhalation and oral. Generally, most of occupational exposure occurs through the dermal route, however the inhalation route may be significant for certain pesticides (e.g. fumigants) and types of pesticide applications (e.g. fogging). Oral exposure to pesticides can result from poor hygiene practices (e.g. smoking and eating with contaminated hands) or from ingestion of inhaled particles trapped in the naso-pharyngeal area.

## PAST

Pesticide exposure assessment is a relatively new field that integrates expertise and knowledge from other established disciplines such as chemistry, toxicology, biology, agronomy and industrial hygiene.

The first efforts to assess occupational exposure to pesticides were triggered by concerns about agricultural workers exposed to acutely toxic organophosphates. This led to the pioneering work by Durham and Wolfe[3]. Prior to their work, only occupational hazard assessments, and not risk assessments, could be conducted. In their classic paper published in 1962 Durham and Wolfe proposed the use of air samples, pads and washes to directly measure exposure to pesticides. In this research, gauze pads in respirators were used to determine airborne concentration of pesticides in the breathing zones of workers. The use of this modified respirator had the advantage of the worker producing the airflow for trapping the pesticide thus avoiding the need to estimate individual breathing rates. The contamination of workers' skin and clothing was measured from deposition on absorbent gauze pads attached to the workers, clothing. Although refinements have been made to these methods over time, the principles of the techniques are still followed. These methods represent the starting point of pesticide exposure assessment.

It is now recognized that field worker exposure can be of similar magnitude to mixer/loader/applicator exposure and that exposure may occur over the growing season. In response to reported illnesses for workers who reenter pesticide treated areas, researchers have developed approaches to estimate field worker exposure and to determine safe reentry intervals or levels[4,5,6,7,8]. More recently, the use of transfer co-efficients derived from the ratio between foliar dislodgeable residues and dermal deposition has been suggested an approach to estimating field worker exposure[4,6,7].

The toxicity of pesticides is generally assessed from studies that are now conducted in accordance with well established and internationally accepted guidelines. However, there are no internationally harmonized guidelines for conducting exposure assessments. Various organizations prepared guidance documents in the 1970's and 1980's (NACA[9], WHO[10,11], EPA[12]) that are still widely used.

The WHO protocol (1975), which was targeted towards measuring dermal exposure to organophosphorus insecticides, recommended the use of the Durham and Wolfe patch methodology. In 1982 a revised WHO protocol entitled "Field Surveys of Exposure to Pesticides" was designed to assess all classes of pesticides. The amended WHO protocol formed the basis of the U.S. National Agricultural Chemicals Association (NACA) exposure guidelines. These guidelines, like those of the WHO, discuss the need for exposure studies based on use pattern and toxicology of the formulation. In 1986 the

US EPA published their guidelines, "Pesticide Assessment Guidelines, Subdivision U, Applicator Exposure Monitoring". Both US EPA and NACA guidelines contain an overview of the advantages and limitations of the various methodological approaches. Health Canada has also prepared draft exposure assessment guidelines with the goal to making them compatible with currently existing guidelines.

One of the limitations with these different guidelines is that studies have been carried out using various methods and approaches that are not standardized making it difficult to compare results. For example the US EPA recommends the measurement of exposure to an individual over a partial workday, whereas Health Canada recommends measurement of exposure to a worker during a full typical workday. Colleagues have recently published a comparative review of available guideline documents[13]. Harmonized exposure and biological monitoring guidelines were proposed in a workshop held in The Netherlands. A proposed guidance document based on a harmonized approach will be discussed later in this volume.

## PRESENT

There have been a number of interesting developments in the field that have significantly affected the way exposure assessments are done. While passive dosimetry as described by Durham and Wolfe is a relatively crude method to determine potential exposure, it is still widely used. Researchers have developed refinements in passive dosimetry techniques such as the use of whole body dosimeters initially proposed by WHO[11] and the use of personal air samplers instead of area air samplers. The proposed guidance document in this volume recommends the whole body technique which has the advantage over the traditional patch method of not requiring the extrapolation of exposures to body surface areas.

Knowledge of occupational exposure gained from passive dosimetry studies have encouraged research and development into agricultural engineering controls such as closed mixing/loading systems and closed cabs tractors with filtered air, new formulations and improved packaging. The increasing use of water soluble packaging for dry pesticide formulations and development of safer formulations (e.g. gels, dry flowables) are two such advances by pesticide manufacturers that are encouraging and should be commended as major initiatives in product stewardship.

There has also been considerable research into the evaluation of personal protective clothing and equipment for pesticide workers. For example, the results of glove permeation studies funded by US EPA indicate that permeation of active ingredients through glove materials is highly dependent of the permeation of the solvent in the pesticide formulation[14].

A limitation of passive dosimetry methods is that they estimate the amount of pesticide that impinges on the body surface and not the amount absorbed into the body. This has generated significant work in the area of development of methods and protocols for dermal absorption (e.g. US EPA protocol[15]). There is considerable research activity in the area of validation of *in vitro* dermal absorption methods which once fully validated may play a greater role in exposure assessment.

The measurement of absorbed dose is perceived as the principal advantage of biological monitoring over exposure monitoring. Biological monitoring involves the analysis of body fluids and excreta for the pesticide, metabolite or biotransformation products which can provide a quantitative estimate of absorbed dose. Biological monitoring has the advantage of integrating exposure from all possible sources and routes, dermal, inhalation and oral. However, to be used effectively, it is necessary to understand the metabolism and pharmacokinectics of the compound in humans. Due to ethical considerations such information may be difficult to obtain. In most cases extrapolations from animal data are performed based on the assumption that metabolism kinetics are similar between human and animal species.

In recent years we have made significant inroads in our scientific understanding into the pharmacokinetics of some chemicals. Comprehensive metabolic studies on pesticides such as phenoxy herbicides has provided a better understanding of their pharmacokinetics that could be used in risk assessment. These types of studies have confirmed that the metabolic pathway in experimental animals is similar to that in humans for phenoxy herbicides. There continues to be a multitude of chemicals which lack the information on human metabolism. Advances in analytical technology enable some exposure studies in human volunteers at doses lower or similar to those likely to be encountered in the occupational setting. This progress should result in an increase use of biological monitoring to estimate exposure.

One major achievement worthy of note is the development of generic descriptive exposure databases, such as US EPA/Health Canada/NACA database[16] (PHED). The basic assumption underlying the database is that pesticide exposure is primarily a function of physical parameters of application rather than the chemical properties of the pesticide. Furthermore, an expert group is working on a similar European database (Europoem). Another model is currently used in the UK. The UK POEM is a semi-quantitative predictive model based on exposure study data[17]. However, these worker exposure databases are only as good as the underlying data. These databases will encourage the use of a tiered approach to pesticide exposure assessment that is described later in this volume.

Video imaging and fluorescent tracers have been proposed to assess dermal exposure in a non-invasive manner[18,19]. One possible advantage of using this approach is that it allows the participation of individuals such as children without the concerns of exposure to pesticide active ingredients. Furthermore qualitative use of fluorescent tracers can be used to identify exposure patterns, evaluate protective clothing performance and as an educational tool to show workers where exposure has occurred.

The regulation of residential pesticidal use has typically been based on hazard rather than exposure and risk quantification. Concern over health risks associated with exposure to residential pesticides has resulted in the development of methodologies for assessing exposures to pesticides used in and around the home. In particular there has been a focus on measuring dislodgeable residues on various surface types with sampling devices designed to simulate human contact. The National Agricultural Chemicals Association (NACA) recommended the use of "coupons" and wipe sampling to measure dislodgeable residues. Other methods that were designed to remove surface contaminants include the polyurethane foam roller (PUF), Dow Drag Sled and the California Cloth Roller[20,21,22]. Preliminary studies indicate that these three techniques remove surface contaminants with reproducible results, but again their relation to actual surface-to-skin transfer is not known. Currently effort is being directed by US EPA and Health Canada towards developing an understanding of these issues[23].

Adherence to Good Laboratory Practices and effective quality control procedures are now commonplace in most analytical laboratories. However, these principles have only recently been extended to the collection, handling, storage and transport of samples during pesticide exposure studies. Procedures related to field sample collection in particular are necessary to identify any losses which may occur between sampling and analysis. Poor Quality Assurance/Quality Control is the major reason for rejection of worker exposure studies as indicated by US EPA Pesticide Reregistration Rejection Rate Analysis.

As mentioned earlier, when pesticide exposure assessment was in its infancy, the major driving force was the need to assess agricultural exposures to acutely toxic products such as ethyl parathion. Pesticide exposure assessment has now greatly expanded to encompass other classes of pesticides, other toxicology endpoints (e.g. carcinogenicity, reproductive effects, teratogenicity) as well as other uses such as industrial, forestry and residential. In Canada as in other industrialized countries while the major pesticide use is by farmers for agricultural crop protection (88%), other scenarios such as home and garden applications (7%), forestry (3%) and industrial vegetation management (2%) are significant[24].

## FUTURE

More research is required to validate passive dosimetry techniques to provide more confidence in these direct methods of exposure assessment and as a consequence in the database models which are based on passive dosimetry data. Passive dosimetry techniques remain largely unvalidated even though they have been used for over 30 years. Biological monitoring and passive dosimetry can also be used to provide realistic estimates of the protective value of personal protective clothing and equipment and other exposure reduction methods. Side by side comparisons would be useful in validating the results from studies using alternative techniques. This would provide more confidence in the use of indirect exposure assessment methods.

The development of physiologically-based pharmacokinetic (PBPK) models shows great promise as means of improving estimates of risk. Although differences in metabolism require that models be specific for a chemical, the anatomical, physiological and biochemical aspects of such models are identical. This has led to research on creating generic PBPK models of animals and humans. Use of these models should allow the prediction and confirmation of the dose delivered to the tissue thus securing more precise exposure and risk assessments. This is important since the relevant tissue dose is not always proportional to external exposure.

A somewhat different approach to biological monitoring is the measurement of biomarkers which is discussed elsewhere in this volume. They are defined as signalling events in biological systems or samples and have been classified as markers of exposure to a toxic substance, markers of effect of exposure and markers of susceptibility to the effects of exposure[25]. The sensitivity, specificity and predictive value of individual biologic markers must be determined for correct interpretation of results. Biomarkers are being recognized as a useful tool in epidemiological studies to supplement traditional methods of exposure evaluation. While biomarkers show great promise, they need further validation before they can be routinely used for regulatory purposes.

While there have been some improvements in engineering controls to reduce exposure not all of these systems are necessarily fail safe and improvements are necessary. There is also a need for more data on which to base any proposed exposure reduction default values provided by various measures and practices such as personal protective clothing penetration e.g. coveralls.

There is a need to develop better methods and guidelines for assessing exposure to workers who reenter treated fields and bystanders who reenter treated residences. At present, information is lacking on dermal transfer coefficients of residues from contaminated surfaces to the skin for specific activities. Furthermore, the removal of residues from surfaces by skin contact requires an understanding of human behaviour patterns. There is a need for the characterization and quantification of activity patterns of occupants such as small children in order to determine the surface areas typically contacted. This information, along with the transfer coefficient, would provide a measure of how much residue is likely to be dermally deposited. The US EPA Subdivision K guidelines[26] on reentry exposure are currently under revision. Considerable research into the area of indoor occupant exposure assessment is either underway or planned by US EPA and Health Canada[24].

Conventional exposure estimates are based on default point estimate parameters (e.g: application rate, dermal absorption, body weight, etc.) that represent a "typical" or "worst-case" value. Exposure evaluators use these point estimate parameters for exposure estimates because of the lack of knowledge or comfort with the quantitative methods used to derive these parameters[27]. Due to the inherent variability there is considerable uncertainty associated with these point estimate parameters of exposure. The use of standard default assumptions for exposure parameters frequently does not produce exposure estimates that represent the exposures experienced in the population[28]. Random number-based techniques account for the uncertainty and variability in the input parameters by combining distributions of exposure parameters stochastically to generate a distribution of exposures. Numerical methods such as Monte Carlo simulations have been used to assess public health risks and are recently being applied to exposure assessment.

Although the main focus of this paper has been on exposure assessment, one should not overlook the impact of various risk mitigation measures (e.g. changes in formulation, personal protective equipment, engineering controls) under actual field use conditions. A good understanding of the protective value of these measures is critical since this is sometimes the only practical way to reduce exposure to pesticides.

The importance of education and training of pesticide applicators as a major vehicle to ensure the safe use of pesticides is being increasingly recognized. Education should result in reduced exposure and risks to applicators and bystanders. In Canada, for example, we are working with provinces to develop a National Standard for Pesticide Education to standardize pesticide applicator programs across the country. The objective of this program is to establish minimum knowledge requirements for all certified applicators through comprehensive and consistent training courses. In a related area, Health Canada conducted a phone survey of corn and apple producers on pesticide use and their attitudes towards safe practices[29,30]. Results indicate that most applicators stated that they wear the minimum protective clothing of pants, long-sleeve shirts and a hat during mixing and loading. Only 31% of corn growers wore chemical resistant gloves compared to 70% of apple growers. Spouses, chemical dealers, farm organizations and farm newspapers were cited as those who most often encourage farmers to wear protective clothing. About half of those surveyed were unaware that following label directions are mandatory and enforceable under Canadian law. A Saskatchewan survey reported that 84% usually or always wear protective gloves while 76% read the product label[31]. More emphasis should be placed on providing pertinent information to the general public and workers on the safe use of pesticides.

## CONCLUSION

This paper has provided an overview of the past, present and some glimpse at the future for the field of exposure assessment. If the goals of the workshop are met, the quality of exposure data that are collected globally should improve thus providing increased protection of the pesticide worker.

## ACKNOWLEDGEMENTS

The authors would like to thank Sesh Iyengar, Pat Curry, Chris Norman and Mary Mitchell for their valuable comments.

## REFERENCES


1. Statistics Canada, "Census Overview of Canadian Agriculture: 1971-1991", catalogue 93-348, May (1992).
2. Anon, A look at world markets, *Farm Chemicals*, pp. 26, 29, 30, 32, 34, September (1985).
3. W.F. Durham and H.T. Wolfe, Measurement of the exposure of workers to pesticides, *Bull. WHO* 26:75-91 (1962).
4. W.J. Popendorf and J.T. Leffingwell, Regulating OP pesticides for farmworker protection, *Residue Rev.* 82:125-201 (1982).
5. H.N. Nigg and J.H. Stamper, Dislodgeable residues of chlorobenzilate in Florida citrus: worker re-entry implications, *Chemosphere* 13:1143-1156 (1984).
6. W.F. Serat, Calculation of a safe reentry time into an orchard treated with a pesticide chemical which produces a measurable physiological response, *Arch. Environ. Contam. Toxicol.* 1:170-181 (1973).
7. W.F. Serat, D.C. Mengle, H.P. Anderson, E. Kahn and J.B. Bailey, On the estimation of worker entry intervals into pesticide treated fields with and without the exposure of human subjects, *Bull. Environ. Contam. Toxicol.* 13:506-512 (1975).
8. R. Krieger, C. Blewett, S. Edmiston, D. Fong, D. Gibbons, L. Meinders, J.R. O'Connell, F. Schneider, J. Spencer and T. Thongsinthusak, Gauging pesticide exposure of handlers (mixers/loaders/applicators) and harvesters in California agriculture, *Med. Lav.* 81:474-479 (1991).
9. NACA, National Agricultural Chemicals Association, "Guidelines for Conducting Biological Monitoring — Applicator Exposure Studies", NACA, Washington, DC (1985).
10. World Health Organisation, Survey of exposure to organophosphorus pesticides in agriculture, Standard protocol, VBC/75.9, WHO, Geneva (1975).
11. World Health Organization, Field surveys of exposure to pesticides, Standard Protocol, VBC/82.1, WHO, Geneva (1982).
12. U.S. Environmental Protection Agency, "Pesticide Assessment Guidelines, Subdivision U, Applicator Exposure Monitoring", U.S. EPA, Washington, DC (1986).
13. P. Curry and S. Iyengar, Comparison of exposure assessment guidelines for pesticides, *Rev. Environ. Contam. Toxicol.* 129:79-93 (1992).
14. A.D. Schwope, Permeation resistance of glove materials to agricultural pesticides, *Am. Ind. Hyg. Assoc. J.* 53(6):352-361 (1992).
15. R.P. Zendzian, Skin penetration method suggested for Environmental Protection Agency Requirements, *J. Am. Coll. Toxicol.* 8(5):829-835 (1989).
16. Health and Welfare Canada, U.S. Environmental Protection Agency, National Agricultural Chemicals Association, Pesticide Handlers Exposure Database (PHED) (1992).
17. C. Lunchick, P. Hamey and S. Iyengar, The use of the North American (PHED) and United Kingdom (POEM) worker exposure models in pesticide registration, Brighton Crop Protection Conference (1994).
18. R.A. Fenske, J.T. Leffingwell and R.C. Spear, A video imaging technique for assessing dermal exposure - I Instrument design and testing, *Am. Ind. Hyg. Assoc. J.* 47:764-770 (1986).
19. R.A. Fenske, S.M. Wong, J.T. Leffingwell and R.C. Spear, A video imaging technique for assessing dermal exposure - II Fluorescent tracer testing, *Am. Ind. Hyg. Assoc. J.* 47:771-775 (1986).
20. J.P. Hsu, D.E. Camann, H. Scattenberg, B. Wheeler, K. Villalobos, M. Kyle, S. Quarderer and R.G. Lewis, New dermal exposure sampling technique, *in:* "Proceedings of EPA/AWMA Conference: Measurement of Toxic and Related Air Pollutants", Durham, NC (1993).
21. J.R. Vaccaro and R.J. Cranston, Evaluation of dislodgeable residues and absorbed doses of chlorpyrifos following indoor broadcast application of chlorpyrifos-based emulsifiable concentrate, Internal Report, Dow Chemical Co., Midland, MI (1990).
22. J. Ross, H.R. Fong and T. Thongsinthusak, Measured potential dermal transfer of surface pesticide residue generated from indoor fogger use: using the CDFA roller method, *Chemosphere* 22:297 (1991).
23. US EPA, Workshop on the Development of Post Application Exposure Monitoring and Assessment Guidelines for Pesticides and Consumer Use Products in Residential Environments, US EPA Report, December 14-15 (1992).
24. Pest Management Alternatives Office, "Feasibility Study for a National Pesticide Use Database", (1994).

25. J.S. Gift, R. Grissom and J.M. Straight, Biological Markers: Monitoring populations exposed to hazardous substances, *J. Environ. Health* 54(2):22-26 (1991).
26. U.S. EPA, "Pesticide Assessment Guidelines, Subdivision K - Exposure: Reentry protection", Adams JD, EPA 540/9-84-001, Washington, DC (1984).
27. G. Whitmyre, J. Driver, M. Ginevan, R. Tardiff and S. Baker, Human exposure assessment I: Understanding the uncertainties, *Toxicol. Indust. Health* 8(5):297-320 (1992).
28. G. Whitmyre, J. Driver, M. Ginevan, R. Tardiff and S. Baker, Human exposure assessment II: Quantifying and reducing the uncertainties, *Toxicol. Indust. Health* 8(5):321-342 (1992).
29. Health and Welfare Canada, "Report on the Findings of a Survey to Assess Apple Growers' Attitudes, Beliefs, Knowledge, and Practices Regarding Pesticide Use", Internal Report (1992).
30. Health and Welfare Canada, "Report on a Survey of Pesticide Application and Safety Practices Among Corn Producers in Ontario and Quebec", Internal Report (1989).
31. L. Dahlgren, S. Marshak and H. McDuffie, Farm family wellbeing survey, Conference on Agricultural Safety and Rural Health, Regina, Saskatchewan (1992).

# PESTICIDE EXPOSURE AND RE-ENTRY IN AGRICULTURE

Joop J. van Hemmen, Yvette G.C. van Golstein Brouwers,
and Derk H. Brouwer

Department of Occupational Toxicology
TNO Nutrition and Food Research Institute
P.O. Box 5815
2280 HV Rijswijk, The Netherlands

## INTRODUCTION

For risk evaluation one needs to know the toxicity of the compound and its uses, since the actual use pattern determines the level of exposure. This is the case for the mixing, loading and application of pesticides, as well as for re-entry exposure, *i.e.* exposure after application. For the present overview the emphasis is on the various aspects of the exposure of harvesters and other workers in a crop. The level of exposure caused by re-entry is determined by the amount available in the surroundings of the worker, *i.e.* the amount present in air (still available after application as vapour and/or aerosols, or available by evaporation from crop, soil, objects, or materials present), or brought into the air by the workers activities (*e.g.* resuspension of deposited residues) and the degree of contact of the worker with contaminated surfaces (mainly the crop itself). The resulting potential exposure, defined as the amount that reaches the worker from the environment by deposition, contact or inhalation, is very important for generic purposes. The potential exposure may be determined by the chemical properties of the pesticide but it is certainly determined by the physical parameters related to the type of crop, physical properties of the pesticide and the nature of the operations of the worker. The major advantage of the concept of potential exposure is given by the fact that the actual clothing of the worker has no influence on the potential exposure. This is, however, also its major disadvantage since for the assessment of systemic uptake of the pesticide through the skin, by inhalation or by swallowing, the actual exposure and the degree of absorption must be known. The actual skin exposure is defined as the amount that reaches the skin and becomes therefore available for absorption through the skin. For inhalation and oral exposure, the potential and actual exposure are (without respiratory protective equipment) generally much more similar than for dermal exposure.

*Methods of Pesticide Exposure Assessment*, Edited by
P.B. Curry *et al.*, Plenum Press, New York, 1995

The most elaborate method for the determination of the absorbed dose is biological monitoring. This method requires, however, a basic pharmacokinetic knowledge of the active ingredient and is therefore compound-specific. The use of biological monitoring, as well as biomarkers or biological effect monitoring for the estimation of risk, it is not considered here further.

In this paper the various experimental and conceptual approaches of re-entry exposure, *i.e.* after application, will be presented, taking the harvesting of ornamentals in greenhouses as an illustration. In recent, as yet unpublished, papers by Mitchell et al., (1993) and Van Hemmen (1993), various aspects of re-entry exposure assessment have been covered as well.

## RE-ENTRY AND EXPOSURE, CONCEPTS AND EXPERIMENTAL EVIDENCE

The term 're-entry' relates to the work activities that concern the entering of an enclosed space and/or a crop after treatment with a pesticide. The detrimental effects of re-entry exposure to workers were noted in the early fifties right after the introduction of parathion and have since been studied in detail, especially in California for organophosphorous compounds (Maddy et al., 1990). The major crops under study were citrus, other tree crops (oranges, peaches, etc.), grapes and cotton. A number of outbreaks of illnesses in California has led to the introduction of re-entry intervals in the USA. The re-entry interval[1] (minimum time period between pesticide application and work activities in the crop, such as harvesting) was largely based on the occurrence of these outbreaks. The largest time periods were set in California, almost all for organophosphorous compounds (Nigg 1980). Popendorf (1992) has recently presented a detailed list of formal re-entry intervals and a thorough analysis of their experimental and theoretical basis.

For prediction purposes a concept was developed in which the primary source of the exposure was the residue of the pesticide. From measurements it was noted that the residues on foliage decayed in time, although sometimes inconsistently (Gunther et al., 1977). The experimental data using measurements for the residues on foliage and on dust particles indicated that oxygen-analogues of thio-organophosphorous compounds were formed on the crop. The importance for the health risk to workers of these findings is the much more toxic nature of the degradation products. The major experimental work was carried out by groups around Gunther, Ware, Knaak, Iwata, Serat, Spear, Spencer, Nigg, and last but not least Popendorf. This work has led to the concept of 'safe levels of dislodgeable residues'.

In the eighties, Popendorf published what he called the 'unified field model'. The concept of this model is presented in Figure 1 in a slightly adapted form. The 'unified field model' has been worked out in detail by Popendorf and Leffingwell (1982) and Popendorf (1985; 1992) for cholinesterase-inhibiting pesticides, but can be adapted to pesticides with other health effects.

### Application and Decay of Pesticide

The purpose of the application of a pesticide to a crop is generally to cover the

[1] The re-entry interval should not be confused with the pre-harvest interval. The first is meant to protect the worker from risks by dermal, inhalation and oral exposure due to surface residues on foliage of the crop, whereas the second is meant to protect the consumer from risks by ingestion of residues in edible commodities.

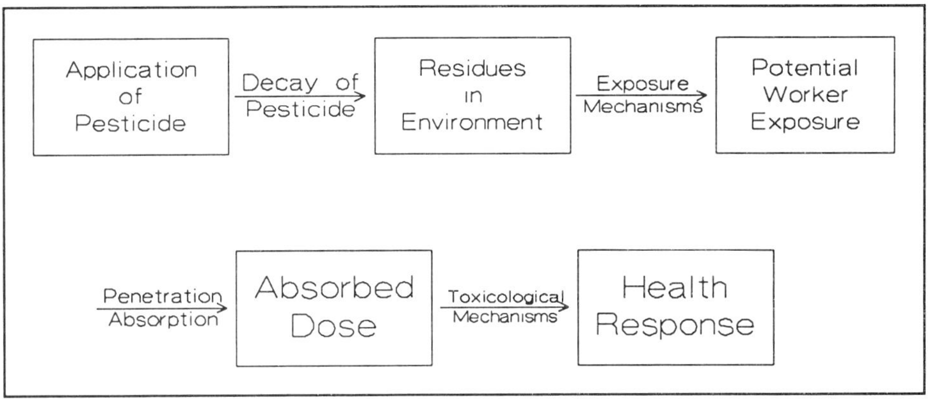


**Figure 1.** The 'unified field model' (adapted from Popendorf, see text).

entire crop. The amount of pesticide is determined by the efficacy for the disease on the crop to be treated or to be prevented. This may be determined by the application rate (*e.g.* kg active ingredient (a.i.) per ha) or by a concentration of the spray liquid. Although the last format is not indicative of the total amount of pesticide per acreage, it may be useful for the farmer in the sense that small (young) crops may need less spray liquid than large (mature) crops. Based on this maximum amount and the leaf area index[2] the amount per surface area of the crop foliage can be estimated. However, quite large variations due to imperfect spraying and incomplete coverage may occur. Especially in the case of low-volume and ultra-low-volume spraying techniques the deposition of the mist on the crop foliage may be appreciably lower than 100% of the applied amount, due to drift (outdoors) and impaction on the walls or elsewhere (indoors). It should be noted that substantial amounts may reach the soil, depending on the size and density of the crop and the technical skills of the applicator. The use of a leaf area index is therefore an approximation of reality.

The health-related problems in California, indicated above, appear to be related to the very dry climate and the dustiness due to work activities. This has been described as 'workers dusted or bathed in dilute residues practically from head to foot' (Quinby and Lemmon 1958). These dust particles may have contained appreciable amounts of pesticide during harvesting. It is therefore important to estimate the decay of the pesticide which eventually leads to the levels of the environmental residues at re-entry. It is further evident from published studies that the decay is determined by many factors, amongst which are the chemical nature of the compounds present, the degree of uptake by the crop, the effects of weathering and decomposition (sunlight, rain, wind and temperature), as well as surface characteristics of the foliage (Ebeling 1963; Willis and McDowell 1987; Bates 1990). As indicated above, the active ingredient may be hydrolysed to a more toxic metabolite as is the case for many thio-organophosphorous compounds such as parathion. It is therefore very important to know or to estimate the decay with time of the active ingredient and its possible metabolites on the foliage and the soil, in case this is relevant for the exposure of the worker. In some cases this decay is very fast, while in other cases, no appreciable decay even over periods of more than weeks has been observed. The form of the decay curve may vary appreciably, although many authors indicate a first order decay as a good approximation of at least the initial

[2] The 'leaf area index' is defined as the total foliage (one-sided) surface area of a crop divided by the ground surface area on which the crop grows.

part. In some cases the kinetics may follow a more complex curve (*e.g.* showing three different half-lives). Stamper et al., (1979) proposed power equations as a more adequate description of the decay. Timme et al., (1986) have fitted decay curves with various mathematical models and investigated their own data sets on 'total residues'. For 420 series the first order model was stated to provide the best fit in 35% of the series and the first order root function to provide the best fit for an additional 35%. The decay of a specific active ingredient may vary with the season of the year and with the geographical region. When no data or estimates are available on the decay of the specific pesticide on the specific crop, absence of decay may be considered a 'worst case'.

**Residues in the Environment and Worker Exposure Mechanisms**

According to recent research there appears to be a rather good correlation between the exposure of the workers and the amount of pesticide on the foliage for crop-workers. This seems to be true for inhalation as well as dermal exposure, although the experimental evidence is by far the strongest for the dermal exposure. The inhalation exposure concerns that part of the particles that reach the alveoli, which therefore must be very small. However, a part of the larger-sized particles may deposit in mouth and upper respiratory tract. This material may be transported to the mouth, swallowed and thus contribute to the oral dose. The dermal exposure of interest is that part of the contamination which reaches the skin by direct contact or deposition on the skin, by penetration through the clothing, or by movement through openings or around the seams of the clothing. Harvesting in wet crops, *e.g.* just treated with pesticides or wet again after rainfall or dew in the morning, may increase the level of exposure.

In the seventies, several investigators have used the occurrence of a biological effect to determine health risks. Especially cholinesterase inhibition for organophosphorous compounds was used. Serat et al., (1975) developed a method to estimate a re-entry interval using such data. Although the implicit notion of linearity between the level of residue and cholinesterase inhibition has turned out to be largely correct, their analysis did not consider exposure influencing variables, like work methods.

For dermal exposure due to contact with the crop, a source strength term is needed, which indicates the availability (dislodgeability) of the pesticide residue on the foliage. There has been some controversy whether the methods for estimating the so-called dislodgeable foliar residues are sufficiently reproducible for different combinations of crop and pesticide. Presently, the method worked out by Iwata et al., (1977) seems to be the most popular one, although minor adaptations are made by various investigators (such as the foliage sampling using leaf punches or whole leaves; this has been discussed by Dong et al., (1991). In this method the amount of pesticide on a leaf surface is 'washed off' with a mild detergent solution to mimic the contact between worker and foliage. For use in the field, kits need to be developed to estimate the dislodgeable foliar residue, in case re-entry is needed and health risks cannot be excluded otherwise.

Several attempts have been made to determine a transfer factor (coefficient) for the estimation of dermal exposure from the level of dislodgeable foliar residue. Popendorf has investigated the relationship between residue and dermal exposure for various studies. From these data (summarized by Popendorf and Leffingwell 1982) it is obvious that there is a linear relationship between these variables over a broad range of values, although the ratio may differ between crops and depend on the work practices. The approach by Popendorf and Leffingwell was also taken and developed further by Nigg et al., (1984) and by Zweig et al., (1985). These authors have studied the relationship between dislodgeable residue on foliage and (in most cases) the total potential dermal exposure to the harvesters for several crops. The observed average ratios[3] vary with values as low as about 800 up to as high as 61,000 $cm^2/hr$ (Zweig et al., 1985). The average value for all studies was about 5,000 $cm^2/hr$ (one-side projection of the leaf-area). This empirical factor was proposed by Nigg et al., (1984) as well, to be used for the estimation of dermal exposure from dislodgeable residue data without the actual measurement of human exposure. A need for further validation using other crop/pesticide combinations was expressed by Zweig et al., (1985).

More recently, Krieger et al., (1990; 1992) have presented transfer factors varying (averaged per study) from about 1,000 to 400,000 $cm^2/hr$ for various harvesting activities. These data were taken from the work of the Worker Safety and Health Branch (California Dept. of Pesticide Regulation). The notion of these authors is that the role of plant contact and work tasks are more important than was initially anticipated. They have considered the various activities on the basis of the actual body contact with the crop. This breaks down from 'sort and select' (only hand contact) to 'expose, search, reach and pick' (full body contact). A further note of caution is given by the fact that the role of time in transferability requires further evaluation, especially for unexpectedly low or high levels of dislodgeable foliar residues. Peelen, Brouwer and Van Hemmen (unpublished results) noted a decrease in transfer rate of chlorothalonil residues over a period of twelve days for the picking of chrysanthemum cutlings. In view of the unknown importance of the chemical nature of the pesticide, the foliage surface, and moisture on the transfer factor the data collected so far should be considered as indicative values. Further evaluation of the available literature is strongly suggested, as is also indicated by Mitchell et al., (1993). The indicative transfer factors cf. Krieger et al. are presented in Figure 2.

**Penetration through Clothing and Skin Absorption**

There is a considerable lack of data concerning the degree of penetration through clothing, since in agricultural practice one is dealing with residues which may be wiped from the foliage by contact or which dislodge due to work activities and deposit as solid aerosols. In hot climates, which may occur both in open air and in greenhouses, the penetration of the solid pesticide (partly adhered to dust particles) may be increased due to the dampening of the clothing by sweating (Raheel 1991) and by crop juices. Several studies are available on the protective capacity of normal clothing and of specially designed protective clothing. In view of the large differences in work practice, climatic conditions and the large variation in clothing, it is difficult to estimate default values which can be used for the degree of protection in a general case. Furthermore the largest body of work is aimed at the mixer/loader and the applicator. For re-entry situations it is evident that the distribution of the contamination will vary largely with the type of crop that is harvested and the type of work. Zweig et al., (1985) have shown *e.g.* that harvesters of strawberries, growing on ground level, were exposed mainly on the hands, whereas weeders in the same crops, who created dusty surroundings, were mainly exposed on the torso.

A major problem in estimating the relevant level of uptake through the skin is the skin absorption itself (Grandjean 1990). Recently, Fiserova-Bergerova (1993) attended this problem. Dermal absorption is affected by the physico-chemical properties of the compound, the variations in the skin, and external conditions which determine the skin

---

3 The units of the ratio (transfer factor) are area per time. The area may be indicative for the lowest amount of foliage surface in $cm^2$ with which the worker comes into contact during an hour with total transfer of the pesticide.

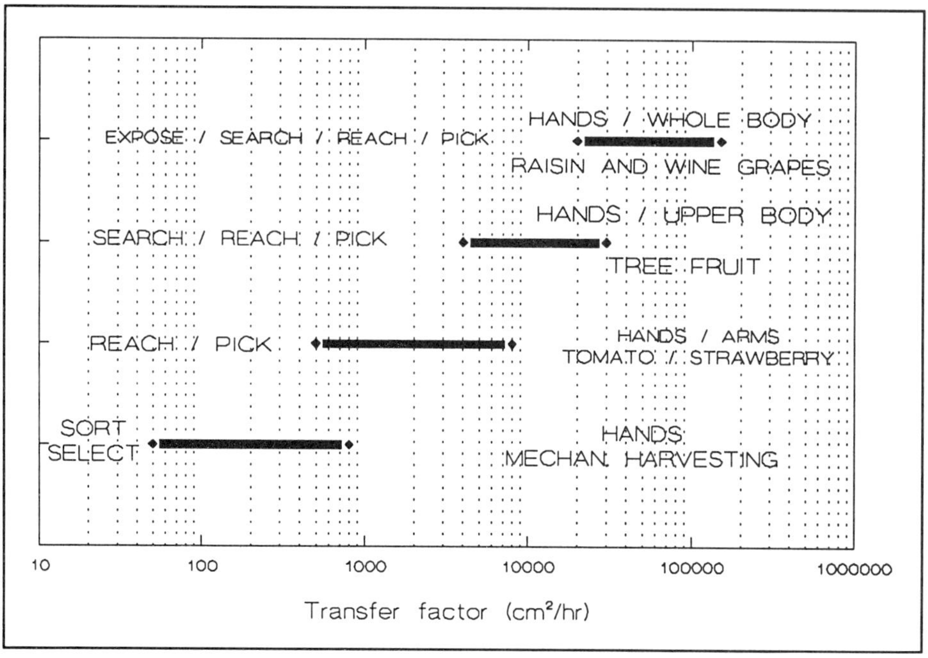


**Figure 2.** Indicative transfer factors for various crop-handling activities (adapted from Krieger, see text).

load with that chemical. The penetration of the skin can be approximated in terms of Fick's first law, which states that the flux ($mg/cm^2.sec$) is the product of the diffusion coefficient and the concentration gradient over the skin. The major penetration process is by diffusion through the stratum corneum and transfer into capillary blood. Since the skin is regionally different, it is important to know how the contamination is distributed over the body. It is obvious that one needs specific data for the compound under consideration. For practical reasons, a percentage absorption is used in pesticide registration procedures, but there is no theoretical basis for this. It is, however, outside the scope of this paper to consider this matter further.

Without knowledge on the absorption one might use a 'worst case' approach. This may amount to about 30% on the basis of animal experimentation and present knowledge. A possible way to overcome the theoretical and practical problems for estimating the absorbed dose is by using biological monitoring, although this will present other problems, such as the requirement of a thorough pharmacokinetic evaluation of the pesticide under study (Woollen 1993).

## Toxicological Mechanisms and Health Effects

On the basis of the presented data it is clear that for pesticides in actual use, the case of cholinesterase-inhibiting compounds is the best studied one, largely elaborated by Popendorf (Popendorf and Leffingwell 1982; Popendorf 1990 and 1992). In the last paper, a rather complete and thorough analysis is made of the published data on decay of compounds on foliage, as well as of the cholinesterase inhibition, reversion and regeneration. Using such an approach re-entry intervals can be calculated.

Such an elaborate approach, as presented by Popendorf for cholinesterase-inhibiting compounds, is lacking for pesticides with other toxic mechanisms. The main reason for this may be that no acute illnesses in groups of workers have been observed amongst harvesters, apart from skin effects. On the other hand the possibilities of using biological effect monitoring for pesticides other than organophosphorous compounds are, presently, scanty.

The comparison of the daily exposure for non-cumulative toxicants or the integrated dose over relevant periods of time and the accepted dose over similar periods for cumulative toxicants, requires detailed toxicological knowledge, obtained from experimental data using animals or humans. On the basis of the toxicity data, obtained with preferably more than one animal species, a lowest no-observed-effect-level of parent compound and relevant metabolites may be deduced. Using extrapolation and uncertainty factors a no-effect-level for humans may then be estimated. Further, the steepness of the dose-response curve for the first and or most important health effect should indicate the basis for an accepted level of absorption. Since pesticides belong to many different chemical classes, the accepted levels for workers by inhalation and by dermal or oral uptake may vary considerably. A further elaboration of the subject of toxicological mechanisms and effects is outside the scope of this paper.

## RE-ENTRY IN GREENHOUSE CROPS

The literature contains relatively few reports on the levels of exposure during crop activities (virtually limited to harvesting) in greenhouses. The reason for this may be that the agricultural size is relatively small and the use of organophosphorous compounds is less important than for instance in citrus culture. The major crops cultivated in greenhouses are ornamental flowers and edible commodities. The pesticide treatment in the last group is regulated by pre-harvest intervals and residue limits to protect the consumer. This is not the case for ornamentals where export of flowers may require a virtually complete absence of (traces of) diseases, which may lead to relatively high frequencies and rates of application.

### Inhalation Exposure

The exposure to fumigants, such as methyl bromide, is not considered here, since it requires a complete compound-specific analysis. The use of low-volume-misters and fogging equipment will give rise to relatively high levels of small liquid aerosols and vapour in the greenhouse over quite long periods in time (Williams 1978; Williams et al., 1980; Lindquist et al., 1987; Liesivuori et al., 1988; Brouwer et al., 1992[d]; Kangas et al., 1993). It can be concluded from this work that re-entry intervals of eight hours, with during the last two hours complete opening of the windows to ventilate the greenhouse, is sufficient for all pesticides, to ensure safe inhalation levels. In the case of volatile compounds (vapour pressure above 10 mPa at 20 °C), it is advised to open the windows to some extent during the next two days to prevent a build-up of possibly toxic concentrations. When high-volume techniques are used for application, it is considered sufficient to use a re-entry interval of eight hours (for non-volatile pesticides) or one hour with the windows wide open (for all pesticides). These numbers are mainly based on the work of Brouwer et al., (1992[d]).

During harvesting, the worker may be exposed to the volatilized pesticide vapour, although this exposure is generally expected to be very low, when re-entry intervals are as described above. Another source of pesticide may be the dislodging (resuspension in air) of (dust) particles, especially when the crop is treated with a dustable powder. Brouwer et al., (1990; 1993) have shown that also in these cases (observed during harvesting of carnations) the inhalation exposure may be very low, and probably determined by the dislodgeable foliar residue.

## Dermal Exposure

Investigations by Morse et al., (1982) have shown that one should not underestimate the possible risks due to the presence of pesticides, even at relatively long periods after treatment, since on chrysanthemums and carnations imported into the USA through Miami from South and Central America appreciable amounts of various pesticides could be found. Löbel and Schunk (1982) showed that 10-20 days after granule-application of aldicarb to the soil of growing chrysanthemums, the picking of cutlings caused an appreciable cholinesterase inhibition in workers, which was completely absent in a control group using rubber gloves. The dislodgeable foliar residue was not measured and it may be that (metabolites of) aldicarb, as a systemic working compound, stemmed from crop juices, which get to the hands during the picking.

In Finnish greenhouses, especially mevinphos has been studied (Jauhiainen et al., 1992; Kangas et al., 1992; 1993) as used for chrysanthemums and roses. The decay on foliage correlated well with the decrease in the observed dermal exposure over the same time period (two days). The half-life on foliage was given as about 9 hours and the transfer factor as 7,200 $cm^2$/hr. Liesivuori (1988) has estimated the half-lives of some pesticides on roses as being 1-2 days.

In German greenhouses the half-lives of various pesticides on various commodities have been determined by Goedicke (1987; 1988[a]; 1988[b]; 1989) and Goedicke et al., 1989). For methamidophos on gherkins, roses and gerbera's, a transfer coefficient of about 700 $cm^2$/hr was estimated by Goedicke (1989).

In Dutch greenhouses the investigations of Brouwer et al., (1992[a]; 1992[b]; 1992[c]; 1993) and Van Hemmen et al., (1992) were aimed at the determination of transfer factors during the harvesting of roses and carnations for various pesticides, to see whether the data had a strong 'generic power'. It was concluded that the harvesting of roses led to somewhat lower transfer coefficients (with average values for three pesticides during cutting, sorting and bundling of 1,200-6,250 $cm^2$/hr) than for the harvesting of carnations (with average values for four pesticides during cutting of 2,800-10,000 $cm^2$/hr). For the picking of chrysanthemum cutlings the transfer factor was about 400 $cm^2$/hr for two pesticides (Peelen, Brouwer and Van Hemmen, unpublished observations). It should be noted that in this work only the transfer to hands and forearms of the workers was estimated. The application rate was a major determining factor for the level of dislodgeable residue. In the Dutch studies, the decay of several pesticides was observed on chrysanthemums (Peelen, Brouwer and Van Hemmen, unpublished observations). These data vary from less than one day up to seven days. A listing for data observed in European greenhouses is presented by Van Hemmen (1993).

Considering once again the 'unified field model' (Figure 1), one might say that the absorbed daily dose is really a function of a source strength, an activity/crop combination, and the penetration/absorption processes. In the first term the application rate and the leaf area index are important factors and in the second term these are the transfer factor and exposure duration. This leads to the following formula (for an ideal world; in the actual world, one should really use a pseudo leaf area index, indicating deviations from ideality through reasons indicated above):

$$\text{The absorbed daily dose} = 0.01\ (AR : LAI) \times TF \times D \times T \times (0{,}01\ ADR)\ \text{(mg/day)},$$

with an application rate of *AR* kg/ha (= 0.01 AR $mg/cm^2$) applied to a crop, with a (pseudo) leaf area index of *LAI*, and work activities with an indicative transfer factor of *TF* ($cm^2$/hr), a decay factor *D* (determined with an appropriate decay model, *e.g.* first order decay (Dong et al., 1992) at time of harvest, over a period of $T$ (hr)), with an average dermal resorption of $ADR$ (%).

As an illustration, an assessment of exposure for the cutting of carnations will be presented. One might assume for the leaf area index a value of $LAI = 5$. $TF$ may be about 5,000 $cm^2$/hr. The decay factor $D = 1$ (no decay, since the harvesting will occur in many events within 24 hr after application). The harvesting time will be about $T$ = 6 hr. The value for skin absorption is probably below 30 % ($ADR$ = 30). On the basis of these assumptions, the absorbed daily dose (ADD) would be:

$$\text{ADD} = (0.01\ AR : 5) \times 5{,}000 \times 1 \times 6 \times 0.01 \times 30 = 18 \times AR \text{ mg/day.}$$

The acceptability of harvesting carnations with bare hands and forearms (daily practice!) will obviously depend on the application rate ($AR$) and the acceptable daily dose and can therefore be estimated. For $AR$ = 1 kg/ha the accepted (daily) dose for workers, determined from animal toxicology, would have to be higher than 18 mg/day, or above 0.25 mg/kg body weight per day (a male person of 70 kg).

A required re-entry interval may be determined for the case in which the decay is known or can be estimated as the time period sufficient to reach the safe foliar residue level. It should be understood that the presumed safe level is dependent on the crop and the work activities for which the level is estimated (Dong et al., 1992). It is further influenced by the distribution of exposure over the body and the prescribed protective clothing.

## CONCLUSIONS

An approach for the estimation of worker exposure during crop activities after treatment of the crop with pesticides is presented. The quality of the result depends very much on the reliability of the transfer factor, which is determined by crop, work activity, and the decay of the pesticide on the foliage. The leaf area index, together with application technique and crop-specific deposition factors are key elements in estimating the initial amount of pesticide on the crop foliage from the application rate. All these aspects deserve much more investigations. Further work has still to be done to determine the contribution of the contamination over the body in relation to the transfer factor and the possibilities of clothing to protect against the actual deposition on the skin. Especially under hot conditions the design of clothing is very important. These investigations will lead to a much better basis for measures to control the level of exposure after re-entry.

## ACKNOWLEDGEMENTS

The authors like to thank the Dutch Ministry of Social Affairs and Employment for the support for literature studies and experimental work regarding occupational pesticide exposure. In particular Chris Maas and Ad Vijlbrief of the Ministry are gratefully mentioned, as well as the co-workers on these issues at TNO.

## REFERENCES

Bates, J.A.R., 1990, The prediction of pesticide residues in crops by the optimum use of existing data, *Pure Appl. Chem.* 62:337-350.

Brouwer, D.H., Brouwer, R., and Van Hemmen, J.J., 1990, Respiratory exposure to field strength dusts in greenhouses during application and re-entry, *in*: "Book of Abstracts Seventh International Congress of Pesticide Chemistry", H. Frehse, E. Kessler-Schmitz and S. Conway, eds., Vol. III, p. 375, I-UPAC, Hamburg, Germany.

Brouwer, D.H., Brouwer, R., De Mik, G., Maas, C.L., and Van Hemmen, J.J., 1992[a], Pesticides in the cultivation of carnations in greenhouses: Part I - Exposure and concomitant health risk, *Am. Ind. Hyg. Assoc. J.* 53:575-581.

Brouwer, D.H., De Vreede, J.A.F., Ravensberg, J.C., Engel, R., and Van Hemmen, J.J., 1992[d], Dissipation of aerosols from greenhouse air after application of pesticides using a low-volume technique. Implications for safe re-entry, *Chemosphere* 24:1157-1169.

Brouwer, R., Brouwer, D.H., Tijssen, S.C.H.A., and Van Hemmen, J.J., 1992[b], Pesticides in the cultivation of carnations in greenhouses: Part II - Relationship between foliar residues and exposures, *Am. Ind. Hyg. Assoc. J.* 53:582-587.

Brouwer, R., Van Maarleveld, K., Ravensberg, L., Meuling, W., De Kort, W., and Van Hemmen, J.J., 1993, Skin contamination, airborne concentrations and urinary metabolite excretion of propoxur during harvesting of flowers in greenhouses, *Am. J. Ind. Med.* 24:593-603.

Brouwer, R., Marquart, H., De Mik, G., and Van Hemmen, J.J., 1992[c], Risk assessment of dermal exposure of greenhouse workers to pesticides after re-entry, *Arch. Environ. Contam. Toxicol.* 23:273-280.

Chester, G., 1993, Evaluation of worker exposure to, and absorption of, pesticides during occupational use and crop re-entry, *Ann. Occup. Hyg.* 37:509-523.

Dong, M.H., Krieger, R.I., and Ross, J.H., 1992, Calculated reentry interval for table grape harvesters working in California vineyards treated with methomyl, *Bull. Environ. Contam. Toxicol.* 49:708-714.

Dong, M.H., Saiz, S.G., Mehler, L.N., and Ross, J.H., 1991, Determination of crop-specific parameters used in foliar mass to area conversion: I. For selected varieties of grapes, *Bull. Environ. Contam. Toxicol.* 46:542-549.

Ebeling, W., 1963, Analysis of the basic processes involved in the deposition, degradation, persistence and effectiveness of pesticides, *Residue Rev.* 3:35-163.

Fiserova-Bergerova, V., 1993, Relevance of occupational skin exposure, Paper presented during the workshop on Occupational Skin Exposure to Chemical Substances, First International Scientific Conference on Occupational Hygiene in Brussels, 1992, *Ann. Occup. Hyg.* 37:673-685.

Goedicke, H.-J., 1987, Rückstände von Pflanzenschutzmitteln auf Pflanzenoberflächen als Quelle für Intoxikationen und Möglichkeiten der Expositionsnormierung, *Z. ges. Hyg.* 33:339-342.

Goedicke, H.-J., 1988[a], Zum Rückstandsverhalten von Pflanzenschutzmitteln an Pflanzenoberflächen, *Z. ges. Hyg.* 34:279-282.

Goedicke, H.-J., 1988[b], Zum Rückstandsverhalten von pirimiphos-methyl auf Tomaten, Blatt- und Bodenoberflächen im Gewächshaus, *Nahrung* 5:475-480.

Goedicke, H.-J., 1989, Exposition durch Rückstände auf Blattoberflächen nach Anwendung von phosphororganischen Insektiziden im intensiven Apfelanbau, *Z. ges. Hyg.* 35:533-535.

Goedicke, H.-J., Hermes, H., and Wagner, R., 1989, Exposition durch Rückstände auf Pflanzenoberflächen nach Anwendung von Pflanzenschutzmitteln im Gewächshaus, *Z. ges. Hyg.* 35:531-533.

Grandjean, P., 1990, "Skin Penetration. Hazardous Chemicals at Work", Taylor & Francis, London, England.

Gunther, F.A., Iwata, Y., Carman, G.E., and Smith, C.A., 1977, The citrus reentry problem: Research on its causes and effects, and approaches to its minimalization, *Residue Rev.* 67:1-139.

Iwata, Y., Knaak, J.B., Spear, R.C., and Foster, R.J., 1977, Worker reentry into pesticide-treated crops I. Procedure for the determination of dislodgable pesticide residues on foliage, *Bull. Environ. Contam. Toxicol.* 18:649-655.

Jauhiainen, A., Kangas, J., Laitinen, S., and Savolainen, K., 1992, Biological monitoring of workers exposed to mevinphos in greenhouses, *Bull. Environ. Contam. Toxicol.* 49:37-43.

Kangas, J., Laitinen, S., Jauhiainen, A., and Savolainen, K., 1992, Exposure of Workers to Mevinphos in Greenhouses. Poster presented at a workshop on Occupational Skin Exposure to Chemical Substances of the First International Scientific Conference on Occupational Hygiene in Brussels.

Kangas, J., Laitinen, S., Jauhiainen, A., and Savolainen, K., 1993, Exposure of sprayers and plant handlers to mevinphos in Finnish greenhouses, *Am. Ind. Hyg. Assoc. J.* 54:150-157.

Krieger, R., Blewett, C., Edmiston, C., Fong, H., Gibbons, D., Meinders, D., O'Connell, L., Ross, J., Schneider, F., Spencer, J., and Thongsinthusak, T., 1990, Gauging pesticide exposure of handlers (mixer/loader/applicators) and harvesters in California agriculture, *Med. Lav.* 81:474-479.

Krieger, R.I., Ross, J.H., and Thongsinthusak, T., 1992, Assessing human exposure to pesticides, *Rev. Environ. Contam. Toxicol.* 129:1-15.
Liesivuori, J., Lihkkonen, S., and Pirhonen, P., 1988, Re-entry intervals after pesticide application in greenhouses, *Scand. J. Environ. Health* 14, Suppl. 1:35-36.
Lindquist, R.K., Krueger, H.R., and Powell, C.C., 1987, Airborne and surface residues of permethrin after high- and low-volume applications in greenhouses, *J. Environ. Sci. Health* B22:15-27.
Löbel, H., and Schunk, W., 1982, Zur Exposition und Gesundheitsgefährdung der Werktätigen in Gewächshausern durch Rückstände cholinesterasehemmender Pflanzenschutzmittel, *Z. ges. Hyg.* 28:697-699.
Maddy, K.T., Edmiston, S., and Richmond, D., 1990, Illnesses, injuries, and deaths from pesticide exposures in California 1949-1988, *Rev. Environ. Contam. Toxicol.* 114:57-123.
Mitchell, M.F., Iyengar, S., and Curry, P., 1993, Re-entry exposure assessment, manuscript in preparation, Workplace Substances and Pesticides Division, Environmental Health Directorate, Health and Welfare Canada, Ottawa, Canada.
Morse, D.L., Baker, E.L., and Landrigan, P.J., 1979, Cut flowers: A potential pesticide hazard, *Am. J. Public Health* 69:53-56.
Nigg, H.N., 1980, Prediction of agricultural worker safety reentry times for organo-phosphate insecticides, *Am. Ind. Hyg. Assoc. J.* 41:340-345.
Nigg, H.N., Stamper, J.H., and Queen, R.M., 1984, The development and use of a universal model to predict tree crop harvester pesticide exposure, *Am. Ind. Hyg. Assoc. J.* 45:182-186.
Popendorf, W.J., 1985, Advances in the unified field model for reentry hazards, *in*: "Dermal Exposure Related to Pesticide Use. Discussion of Risk Assessment", R.C. Honeycutt, G. Zweig and N.N. Ragsdale, eds., ACS Symp. Series 273:323-340, American Chemical Society, Washington, D.C.
Popendorf, W., 1992, Reentry field data and conclusions, *Rev. Environ. Contam. Tox.* 128: 71-117.
Popendorf, W.J., and Leffingwell, J.T., 1982, Regulating organophosphate residues for worker protection, *Residue Rev.* 82:125-201.
Quinby, G.E., and Lemmon, A.B., 1958, Parathion residues as a cause of poisoning in crop workers, *J. Am. Med. Assoc.* 166:740-746.
Raheel, M., 1991, Pesticide transmission in fabrics: Effect of perspiration, *Bull. Environ. Contam. Toxicol.* 46:837-844.
Serat, W.F., Mengle, D.C., Anderson, H.P., Kahn, E., and Bailey, J.B., 1975, On the estimation of worker entry intervals into pesticide treated fields with and without the exposure of human subjects, *Bull. Environ. Contam. Toxicol.* 13:506-512.
Stamper, J.H., Nigg, H.N., and Allen, J.C., 1979, Organophosphate insecticide disappearance from leaf surfaces: An alternative to first-order kinetics, *Environ. Sci. Technol.* 13:1402-1405.
Timme, G., Frese, H., and Laska, V., 1986, Zur statistischen Interpretation und graphischen Darstellung des Abbauverhaltens von Pflanzenbehandlungsmittel-Rückständen II, *Pflanzenschutz-Nachrichten Bayer* 39:188-204.
van Hemmen, J.J., 1993, Re-entry exposure and product development. Pesticides and greenhouse crops: An example, presented in Brussels, June 1993 at a seminar on Agrochemical Occupational Risk Assessment. The Future, Jellinek, Schwartz & Connolly, Inc., Washington, DC, USA.
van Hemmen, J.J., Brouwer, R., and Brouwer, D.H., 1992, Worker exposure to pesticides in greenhouses. Health risks during harvesting of flowers, *Med. Fac. Landbouww. Univ. Gent.* 57/3b:1269-1283.
Williams, I.H., 1978, Dissipation of sulfotep and nicotine in a greenhouse atmosphere following their use as fumigants, *J. Environ. Sci. Health* B13:235-241.
Williams, D.T., Denley, H.V., and Lane, D.A., 1980, On site determination of sulfotep air levels in a fumigating greenhouse, *Am. Ind. Hyg. Assoc. J.*, 41:647-651.
Willis, G.H., and McDowell, L.L., 1987, Pesticide persistence on foliage, *Rev. Environ. Contam. Toxicol.* 100:23-73.
Woollen, B.H., 1993, Biological monitoring for pesticide exposure, *Ann. Occup. Hyg.* 37(5):525-540.
Zweig, G., Leffingwell, J.T., and Popendorf, Wm., 1985, The relationship between dermal exposure by fruit harvesters and dislodgeable foliar residues, *J. Environ. Sci. Health* B20:27-59.

# Session One

# Guidance Document for the Conduct of Field Studies to Evaluate the Exposure of Operators, Workers, and Bystanders to Pesticides

## SESSION ONE - THE GUIDANCE DOCUMENT

## PREFACE

Session Leader: Dr. Leonard Ritter

Executive Director
Canadian Network of Toxicology Centres
620 Gordon Street
Guelph, Ontario
Canada N1G 1Y4

The goal of session one was to review and revise a draft guidance document on pesticide exposure assessment methods for proposal to the Organisation for Economic Co-operation and Development (OECD). The assessment of occupational exposure to pesticides is an essential component of risk assessment in the evaluation of overall product safety and in the regulatory decision-making process. Today, more than ever before, regulatory officials, industry and users recognize the potential for occupational exposure to pesticides and the need to assess potential health risks which may be associated with this exposure. Similarly, while regulatory officials internationally have accepted their responsibility to consider occupational exposure in the overall assessment of risks, initiatives in international trade and shrinking research budgets have dictated that wherever possible, study protocols, data requirements and approaches to assessment must be harmonized. While guidelines and protocols have been proposed by national regulatory agencies previously, the recent emphasis on the contribution of occupational exposure to overall risk has focused new attention on the need for a unified global approach to the assessment of pesticide exposure.

*Methods of Pesticide Exposure Assessment*, Edited by
P.B. Curry *et al.*, Plenum Press, New York, 1995

## SESSION ONE - THE GUIDANCE DOCUMENT

## RAPPORTEURS' REPORT

Rapporteurs: Margherita Conti[1], and Sylvester Rozario[2]

Health Canada
[1]Toxicological Evaluation Division
[2]Chemical Evaluation Division
Ottawa, Ontario
Canada K1A 0L2

## INTRODUCTION

The session opened with the presentation of a proposed guidance document. The document outlined a harmonized approach for field studies designed to assess pesticide exposure. The document had been circulated to a number of experts who were asked to provide and present a critical analysis of various components of the document. The workshop format then provided an opportunity for discussion of the proposal and critique by the participating international delegates. The presentations and discussion focused on four areas:

* study design
* quality assurance/quality control (QA/QC)
* biological monitoring and passive dosimetry techniques
* ethical considerations

## STUDY DESIGN

Delegates extensively debated the most appropriate sampling period. While most agreed that a "representative day" should include all tasks normally carried out in a day, delegates also recognized that dosimeters may become saturated and need to be replaced. Delegates also expressed the view that it would be inappropriate to monitor only a small portion of the day and extrapolate to a whole day. However, it was indicated that replicates of shorter duration should be considered for volatile and/or unstable compounds.

A sample size of 30 was proposed based on statistical arguments, however, concern was expressed regarding the practical difficulties in disposing of large quantities of treated crop. A sample size of 10 rather than 30 was proposed, recognizing that with

*Methods of Pesticide Exposure Assessment*, Edited by
P.B. Curry *et al.*, Plenum Press, New York, 1995

sample sizes of 10, the mean must be used and not the variance. Sample sizes of less than 10 were generally not considered to be of value.

Delegates acknowledged the potential value of the fluorescent tracer technique and agreed that the guidance document should reflect its potential for the quantification of exposure.

## QA/QC

The discussion on quality assurance/quality control centred on possibilities for reducing the number of QA/QC samples in an exposure study. There was support for using pre-study field recovery data to reduce the requirement for the number of recovery samples. It was agreed that regulators would need to be flexible regarding the number of recovery samples required based on consideration of the physical/chemical properties of the chemical, similarity of environmental conditions and consistency of recoveries in the pre-study.

## BIOLOGICAL MONITORING AND PASSIVE DOSIMETRY TECHNIQUES

There was extensive discussion of the relative strengths and weaknesses of both biological monitoring and passive dosimetry. While some delegates felt that biological monitoring was the best method for estimating exposure, others noted that the strength of this approach was directly related to the availability of appropriate human pharmacokinetic data. It was generally agreed that the use of biological monitoring data must include the consideration of individual variability, genetic disposition and the number of test subjects required to establish statistical validity. In addition, the use of biomarkers should be considered as a potential biomonitoring technique for assessing pesticide exposure.

Concern was expressed that significant differences have been reported between biological monitoring and estimates of internal dose resulting from passive dosimetry. These discrepancies may be due to differences in trapping efficiencies of passive dosimeters and skin, as well as the undetected contribution of additional routes of exposure (i.e. oral) when using conventional passive dosimetry techniques.

Recognizing that the hands often receive the majority of dermal exposure, delegates had a lively exchange on the relative merits of utilizing the hand glove monitoring method when compared to the hand rinse method. A comparison of the two methods was recognized as an area for future research.

Discussion on passive dosimetry also included a review of whole body dosimetry and its practical limitations in developing countries. A whole body wash technique was identified as a possibility for situations where other passive dosimetry methods were not feasible.

## ETHICAL CONSIDERATIONS

There was a general discussion regarding the use of humans in field exposure studies and controlled human pharmacokinetic studies. Concern was expressed about the ethical and human rights considerations. However, delegates recognized that much of the concern originated from a poor understanding within the community regarding the conduct of such studies, and the need to promote better understanding. There was general agreement that the guidance document should address the issues associated with the conduct of human studies, and ensure that the document be available to the general public.

## SUMMARY OF KEY AREAS OF REVISION

The session concluded with the identification of eight key areas of the proposed guidance document which required revision. These included:

i) The duration of the sampling period should be representative of a typical working day. This will ensure that all the work activities which result in exposure, including equipment repair and cleanup are monitored. Biological monitoring studies, in particular, should involve monitoring over the complete working day. Replicates of shorter duration would be considered for volatile and/or unstable compounds.

ii) A section will be added on study design for post-registration surveillance. There was unresolved discussion as to whether these surveillance studies would be used for measuring exposure under actual conditions, for validating the label, or as a compliance tool.

iii) Consideration will be given to reducing the number of QA/QC samples required. This will be based on pre-field studies, previously generated recovery data, physical/chemical properties, ambient conditions and selective sample analysis.

iv) The QA/QC section will be expanded and moved into an Appendix.

v) A description of the fluorescent tracer technique will be added which will include more detail on its quantitative use and limitations.

vi) The "refined whole body dosimeter" method will be further described and will explain the calculation of potential and actual dermal exposure.

vii) An annex will be added providing more detail on passive dosimetry and biological monitoring methodologies. The draft Canadian Guidelines on Pesticide Exposure and the United States Environmental Protection Agency's Pesticide Assessment Guidelines, Subdivision U, Applicator Exposure Monitoring will be used as the basis for this expansion.

viii) The reference to the modified respirator for inhalation monitoring will be removed.

# THE CONDUCT OF FIELD STUDIES TO EVALUATE THE EXPOSURE OF OPERATORS, WORKERS, AND BYSTANDERS TO PESTICIDES

Graham Chester

ZENECA Agrochemicals
Stewardship & Safety Department
Fernhurst, Haslemere, Surrey GU27 3JE

## INTRODUCTION

The evaluation of exposure is an integral part of risk assessment for product safety and regulatory assessment purposes. The purpose of this document is to review the rationales for the possible approaches, the available methods of pesticide exposure assessment and to provide guidance on the determination of exposure to, and absorption of, pesticides by operators, workers and bystanders. The assessment of exposure to bystanders in the indoor environment is beyond the scope of this guidance document. A set of guidelines is appended and further detailed information on the proposed methods can be obtained from published guidelines and references given in this document. The guidance may be useful also to those investigators involved in post-registration surveillance or routine monitoring of exposure to pesticides. The guidance is provided essentially for the measurement of exposure and absorbed dose for quantitative risk assessment. It is not intended to cover biological effect monitoring which may be used as an adjunct to exposure or absorbed dose measurement.

## RATIONALE FOR THE NEED FOR GUIDELINES FOR THE CONDUCT OF WORKER EXPOSURE STUDIES

The essential components of a quantitative risk assessment for operators, workers and bystanders are a detailed evaluation of the toxicity of the compound, the likelihood of the expression of any toxicological effect in humans and an estimation or measurement of the exposure and/or amount absorbed by humans as a consequence of its use. The evaluation of the toxicity of new pesticides is conducted according to internationally accepted guidelines using harmonized methods and protocols. For the best possible risk assessment the evaluation of exposure ought to be equally standardized using harmonized methods and protocols. At present there is no such internationally accepted, harmonized approach to this evaluation.

*Methods of Pesticide Exposure Assessment*, Edited by
P.B. Curry *et al.*, Plenum Press, New York, 1995

Guidelines and Standard Protocols have been published previously and notable examples are the WHO Standard Protocol and the U.S. EPA Guidelines on applicator/operator exposure (WHO, 1982; U.S. EPA, 1986). Since their publication there has been a marked shift in emphasis in regulatory risk assessment in several countries to take account of the extent of occupational exposure and, in particular, the absorbed dose of the compound. This has led to the development of more sophisticated approaches and methods, notably the increasing use of biological monitoring to measure the extent of absorption of pesticides interpreted with the aid of pharmacokinetic data from human volunteer studies. This has developed from the traditional use of biological effect monitoring to assess health effects or modification of normal biochemical indices in workers. There is therefore a need to draw together and review the available methods and present a harmonized approach.

## GLOSSARY OF IMPORTANT TERMS

### Ambient Exposure Monitoring

(1) 'Potential dermal exposure' - the total amount of pesticide coming into contact with the protective clothing, work clothing and the skin.

(2) 'Actual dermal exposure' - the amount of pesticide coming into contact with bare (uncovered) skin and the fraction penetrating the protective and work clothing to the underlying skin, and which is therefore available for percutaneous absorption.

(3) 'Inspirable fraction' of airborne particulate - that fraction capable of entering the respiratory tract via the nose and the mouth, so providing a source of absorption into the body, either from direct inhalation or from subsequent oral ingestion.

### Biological Monitoring

Measurement of a pesticide or its metabolites in the body fluids of exposed persons and conversion to an equivalent absorbed dose of the pesticide based on a knowledge of its human metabolism and pharmacokinetics (Woollen, 1993).

## REVIEW AND COMPARISON OF METHODOLOGY

### Previous Reviews

Early extensive reviews of methodology were by Durham and Wolfe (1962), Wolfe (1976) and Davis (1980). These reviews, and particularly the methodology of Durham and Wolfe (1962), formed the basis of the World Health Organisation (WHO) standard protocol for the measurement of exposure (WHO, 1975; 1982). The first WHO protocol (1975) was aimed primarily at the measurement of exposure to, and absorption of, organophosphorus insecticides and included the Durham and Wolfe 'patch' methodology to estimate dermal exposure. The revised protocol of 1982 was designed to assess all classes of pesticide together with an alternative method for the measurement of dermal exposure (the 'whole body' clothing technique) and an overview of biological monitoring as a means of measuring absorption arising from all routes of exposure. This revised protocol formed the basis of the US National Agricultural Chemicals Association (NACA) guidelines for mixer-loader-applicator exposure studies (Mull and McCarthy, 1986). These guidelines placed primary emphasis on the use of the Durham and Wolfe (1962) 'patch' methodology with scant reference to the more recently developed 'whole body' technique which had figured prominently in the WHO protocol of 1982.

In 1985 NACA also published guidelines for the conduct of field biological monitoring studies as a means of measuring the absorption of pesticides (NACA, 1985). Both the EPA and NACA guidelines contained detailed and useful reviews of the advantages and limitations of the various approaches to the measurement of exposure to, and absorption of, pesticides. More recently, the International Group of National Associations of Manufacturers of Agrochemical Products (GIFAP) (now known as the European Crop Protection Association, (ECPA)) published a position paper on broad aspects of monitoring studies in the assessment of worker exposure to pesticides (GIFAP, 1990). These guidelines were intended to inform the non-specialist of the various approaches to exposure/absorption evaluation and their significance. They were not intended to give detailed descriptions of the various monitoring techniques nor to recommend a specific approach.

Curry and Iyengar (1992) reviewed and compared the currently available guidelines (published and unpublished) for the evaluation of exposure to individuals using pesticides and those exposed to residues in indoor and outdoor environments. Harmonized exposure and biological monitoring guidelines (and the tiered approach to evaluation) were proposed in a workshop involving international experts held in The Netherlands (Henderson *et al.*, 1993). The Worker Health and Safety Branch of the California Environmental Protection Agency have published a guidance document on the preparation of pesticide exposure assessment documents (Thongsinthusak *et al.*, 1993). The document gives information on default values for an exposure assessment, such as body surface areas, bodyweights, ventilation rates and clothing protection factors. The facets of the risk assessment process in California are described in detail.

### Methods For Measuring Dermal Exposure

**Patch Method.** In the patch method, the potential contamination of the workers' skin and clothing is measured using a variable number of absorbent cloth or paper patches attached to defined areas of the body, inside and outside clothing. The patches are the so-called "dosimeters" in "passive dosimetry" and act as a collection medium for the pesticide. After a defined or measured period of exposure, the patches are removed and analyzed for pesticide content. In many published studies, a number of patches were used per worker which represented about 8% of the total body area of approximately 2 $m^2$. The quantity of a pesticide on a patch of known area is then related to the area of limb or other body part on the assumption of uniformity of deposition over the body parts. This assumption is perhaps the principal disadvantage of the patch technique. This is illustrated by the extrapolation of the value given by the limit of quantification (LOQ) to the total body part. This may give a substantial under- or over-estimate of exposure. Individual body part exposure values are then added to give a total potential exposure expressed in mg/hour, mg/day or mg/kg product handled or applied. In the WHO protocol fewer patches are recommended, representing only 3% of the body area. In both cases standard body part surface areas are used in correcting individual patch values (Berkow, 1931; Poppendorf and Leffingwell, 1982). According to the WHO Protocol, only the pesticide contacting the normally unclothed area of skin, for example head, neck, hands, forearm, is used to calculate actual exposure. In temperate climates about 10% of the total body area is normally unprotected during use of pesticides and other agricultural activities.

It is still necessary to estimate exposure to the covered areas of the body. Normal work clothing, such as cotton trousers or shirts, is absorbent and may retain a proportion of the pesticide. Consequently the amount of pesticide penetration is often measured using patches attached beneath the clothing. Without such measurements, an estimate of permeation of normal clothing is usually proposed. However, penetration of clothing by pesticides is a highly variable process which is influenced by such factors as the type of formulation (liquid or solid) and the amount or volume of deposition on the clothing, dampness of the clothing, the location of deposition (e.g., seams) and the type of fabric. Further uncertainties are introduced by the method of sampling for clothing penetration.

The patch method may give significant under- or over-estimates of exposure, depending on whether the patches have captured the non-uniform, random deposition of concentrate splashes or spray droplets. Similarly for crop re-entry procedures, such as harvesting, where contact with the crop is not a uniform process. One solution to the problem of non-uniform exposure is an increase in sample size. The development of the Pesticide Handlers Exposure Database (PHED, 1992) is an attempt to give a more accurate estimate of exposures to different body regions.

**Video Imaging/Use of Fluorescent Tracers.** A recent technical advance has been the development of a video imaging/fluorescent tracer technique (Fenske, 1987). This method involved the incorporation of a fluorescent tracer in a pesticide formulation and subsequent visual and quantitative analysis using a video imaging technique. It revealed non-uniform patterns of exposure which escape detection by the patch technique. It also demonstrated that substantial exposure occurs beneath protective clothing. The main limitation of this method is the assumption that permeation of the clothing by the dye and the pesticide are equivalent. However, this can be corrected if the permeation of the dye and the pesticide are known. The technique does not offer a clear advantage over addition of a dye or other form of tracer to the pesticide formulation or spray tank followed by visual and quantitative analysis. Both suffer from the same limitation. However, the techniques are particularly useful for the training of operators.

**Whole Body Method.** One means of overcoming the inherent problems of the patch method is the use of lightweight protective coveralls or similar type of clothing in the whole body method (WHO, 1982; Abbott *et al.*, 1987). This method is more convenient in a practical sense, in that investigators do not need to attach patches to clothing and skin of workers, which is a time-consuming process. Any additional protective clothing and equipment recommended for the product in question are worn over the sampling clothing, thus enabling an evaluation of their protection. The use of the whole body method overcomes the perceived problem of non-uniformity of deposition in that, if protective materials are used as the sampling medium, most of the pesticide is likely to be captured. Furthermore, extrapolation from small target areas to larger body regions is not necessary. For these reasons, the method is believed to give a more accurate estimate of potential dermal exposure, although it is recognized that it is not possible at present to validate this perceived accuracy.

A variation of the method involves cotton undergarments (long pants and long-sleeved 'T' shirts) worn beneath the normal work clothing to estimate dermal exposure on the entire part of the body covered. This method may be useful for low use rate preparations which can be predicted to have levels of contamination below the limit of quantification applicable to the patch technique.

A refinement of the whole body method is the use of work clothing which represents what the workers would normally wear under the prevailing conditions (Chester *et al.*, 1990). An advantage of this method is that the capture and retention properties of the normal work clothing are mimicked as closely as possible. The method is particularly useful when concurrent exposure and biological monitoring are to be carried out. This adaptation overcomes one of the major criticisms of the patch and standard whole body methods, which is that by putting exposure sampling media or 'barriers' between the pesticide and the clothing or skin, the normal process of contamination and percutaneous absorption is interfered with, thus preventing a representative measurement of absorption.

This method is particularly relevant for North European and North American temperate countries where the typical work clothing consists of a 'T' shirt, long sleeved shirt, socks and long trousers and/or coveralls. Such clothing may also be relevant for some tropical countries. Where measurement of exposure only is undertaken, two coveralls of the same material may be used. Actual exposure of the skin beneath the clothing can be estimated by taking account of the ratio of outer to inner clothing permeation of the pesticide. For analytical considerations, it may be necessary to use non-coloured, white materials such as cotton or cotton/polyester mixtures. The clothing can be sectioned into individual body parts and analysed separately in the same way as the coveralls to determine the regional distribution of, and total potential and actual, exposure.

This method is recommended particularly where it is considered necessary to make a concurrent measurement of absorption using biological monitoring.

It should be noted that little attempt has been made to validate methods for the monitoring of dermal exposure, for example using biological monitoring to compare the derivations of absorbed dose. Until such time, all methods should be regarded as providing only an indicative measure of the dermal exposure. The challenge is to find a sampling medium that mimics skin in its pesticide capture and retention characteristics. Given that biological monitoring for determination of absorbed dose does not lend itself to all pesticides, for example, because of extensive metabolism or routes of elimination other than the kidney, there remains a need to develop and refine exposure methods.

The main advantages and limitations of the methods for estimating dermal exposure are summarised in Table 1.

**Table 1.** Main advantages and limitations of the methods for estimating dermal exposure

| Dermal Exposure Method | Main Advantage | Main Limitation | Use with Concurrent Biological Monitoring |
|---|---|---|---|
| Patch | Ease of analysis | Assumes uniform deposition | Yes (?) |
| Whole body | No body region size or surface area correction necessary | Cumbersome analysis | No |
| Refined whole body | Collects most pesticide not reaching skin | Cumbersome analysis | Yes |
| Dyes/video imaging | Visual and quantitative analysis | Assumes clothing permeation of dye and pesticide equivalent | Yes |

**Hand Exposure.** Monitoring of hand exposure may be the most important measurement in a dermal exposure study. The contribution of the hands to total exposure is well documented. Many investigators, deploying a variety of methods, have demonstrated this contribution (U.S. EPA, 1986). The methods range from the use of lightweight absorbent gloves or sections cut from gloves, swabbing or rinsing the hands in various solvents (U.S. EPA, 1986) to simulating the normal process of washing the hands with soap and water during concurrent biological monitoring (Chester *et al.*, 1990). All these approaches have their advantages and limitations and it is not possible to evaluate the accuracy of any procedure. The best that can be achieved for a handwash method is a laboratory validation of the efficiency of recovery of material from the hands of human volunteers. U.S. EPA (1986) states that the use of gloves may result in a significant over-estimation of total dermal exposure, owing to their capacity to retain more of the pesticide than would otherwise be retained by the skin. Gloves also contain foreign materials, which, unless pre-extracted, may be co-extracted with the pesticide. At low levels of contamination this may be a problem. However, the levels of glove contamination due to dirt and grease are a greater problem in this respect. The hands also tend to incur significant levels of contamination with the pesticide and low level interference may not be as significant a problem as inferred by U.S. EPA (1986).

Washing the hands with a solvent is considered by some to disrupt skin barrier function and enhance percutaneous absorption of the pesticide. U.S. EPA (1986) claim that there is little actual evidence for this and recommend washing using the bag rinse method developed by Durham and Wolfe (1962). Their preference for this technique over washing of the hands in a bowl appears to be because it is a standardized procedure and that the data generated are consistent with those in the existing data base.

In conclusion, it is not possible to recommend one method for estimating hand exposure over another in so far as accuracy of measurement is concerned. The use of a sampling glove is recommended from the stand point of practicability in the field.

Where exposure and absorption measurements are to be conducted concurrently, a washing procedure involving soap and water is proposed for use whenever the workers would normally wash their hands and where it is feasible to do so. The rationale for this proposal is that when absorption is assessed there should be no interference with the normal process of dermal contamination and percutaneous absorption. Therefore the use of absorbent gloves or a solvent washing or rinsing technique is inappropriate, since they would retain pesticide otherwise available for absorption. By performing a handwash with ordinary soap and water, whenever the worker chooses to wash his hands, this normal process of contamination and absorption is not unduly influenced. This technique may provide an estimate of hand exposure, particularly if the worker chooses to wash at frequent intervals such as after mixing or at meal breaks. The major disadvantage is the loss of standardization between workers due to the variable number of handwashes. Any protective gloves worn may also be taken for analysis to determine potential exposure, together with any protective glove washings. An important analytical consideration is the validation of the extraction efficiency of the chosen soap and water prior to the field study. It is recommended that the soap is standardized for all workers in the study to at least ensure consistency of extraction efficiency.

The main advantages and limitations of the methods for estimating the exposure of the hands are summarised in Table 2.

**Table 2.** Main advantages and limitations for estimating the dermal exposure of the hands

| **Hand Exposure Method** | **Main Advantage** | **Main Limitation** | **Use with Concurrent Biological Monitoring** |
|---|---|---|---|
| Absorbent gloves | Ease of use | Possible over-estimation of exposure | No |
| Solvent/swab rinse wash | Standardized method enabling comparison with most previous data | May disrupt barrier function of skin | No |
| Handwash (soap and water) | Does not interfere with process of skin contamination and absorption | Loss of standardization between workers | Yes |

## Methods For Measuring Inhalation Exposure

One of the earlier but most complete reviews of the methodology for field monitoring of airborne pesticides was by Lewis (1976). Van Dyk and Visweswariah (1975) had previously reviewed the media available for collection of pesticides but with particular emphasis on static environmental sampling. A personal air sampling technique is the method of first choice for the determination of airborne concentrations of pesticides in the breathing zones of workers. Several techniques are available ranging from the use of gauze pads in respirators, pioneered by Durham and Wolfe (1962), to solid adsorbents and filter cassettes attached to battery powered personal sampling pumps. The use of the respirator has the principal advantage of the worker producing the airflow for trapping the pesticide and thus circumventing the need for estimation of the breathing rate and total volume of air sampled. A respirator without modification to simulate the nasal orifices will not differentiate between inspirable and non-inspirable material; nor can the fit and seal of the respirator around the face be guaranteed. Use of such a device would also interfere with biological monitoring and would be uncomfortable to wear for long periods, particularly in a hot climate. For these reasons, a personal sampling technique involving sampling devices mounted in the breathing zone and personal sampling pumps is preferred. One problem in the use of sampling pumps is the possible need to change them during long working days due to discharge of the batteries. This necessitates having an ample number of fully charged reserve pumps. Use of the personal air sampler does permit any label-recommended use of respirators or dust masks. The choice of sampling medium is dictated by the nature of the pesticide in that a suitable filter cassette or sampling head should be used for spray particulates and a solid adsorbent material for volatile compounds.

As stated previously, the inspirable fraction (all material capable of being drawn into the nose and mouth) is the most relevant fraction to measure. An example of a suitable personal sampling head is the Institute of Occupational Medicine (IOM) personal sampling head designed specifically to collect this fraction (Vincent and Mark, 1987). For use of this device, a sampling flow rate of 2 l/min is a specific requirement. Examples of suitable adsorbent materials for some volatile compounds are activated charcoal, 'Tenax' and XAD-2 resins mounted in stainless steel or glass tubes. The choice of material should be determined by analytical retention and extractability studies before monitoring.

It may be necessary to sample concurrently for particulates and vapour, in which case the filter sampling head is mounted in front of the vapour trap in a 'sampling train'. This train allows retention of any vapour stripped off the filter on the resin. The material on the filter can be analyzed both gravimetrically and/or chemically and an estimate made of the pesticide content of the particulate sample. Where use of such a sampling train is indicated, laboratory validation of the sampling efficacy, particularly of the adsorbent resin, is necessary owing to the possibility of stripping material from the resin by the relatively high flow rate of 2 l/min.

The measurement of the inspirable fraction and use of adsorbent resins for the vapour component is recommended as the method of first choice.

The advantages and limitations of the methods for estimating the exposure by inhalation are summarised in Table 3.

## Methods For Measuring The Absorbed Dose (Biological Monitoring)

Biological monitoring is a method of evaluating the absorption of chemicals by measuring the chemical or its metabolites in body fluids, usually blood, urine or exhaled breath. Biological <u>effect</u> monitoring has been used in the chemical industry for many years to assess health effects or modification of normal biochemical indices in workers

**Table 3.** Main advantages and limitations of the methods for estimating exposure by inhalation

| Inhalation Exposure Method | Main Advantage | Main Limitation | Use With Concurrent Biological Monitoring |
|---|---|---|---|
| Respirator | Wearer provides own airflow | Discomfort | No |
| Personal air sampler (inspirable/ vapour) | Measures potential inhalation and subsequent oral ingestion | Need to estimate ventilation rate | Yes |

as a consequence of exposure. In the context of pesticides it has been most frequently used for assessing exposure to organophosphorus compounds by measurement of blood cholinesterase activity (see for example, Peoples and Knaak, 1982).

Analysis of body fluids and excreta, most commonly blood and urine, for pesticide or metabolites can provide both a qualitative and a quantitative measurement of absorbed dose. This measurement of absorbed dose is perceived as the principal advantage of biological monitoring over ambient exposure monitoring since it evaluates actual, rather then potential, absorption. It integrates absorption from all possible routes of exposure: dermal, inhalation and primary and secondary oral ingestion. However, it is difficult to differentiate the contributions to the absorbed dose from different aspects of the work, i.e., mixing, loading or application. This can only be done with a specifically tailored study design. For specific details and wider ranging discussions of biological monitoring, the reader is referred particularly to Van Heemstra-Lequin and Van Sittert (1986), Wang *et al.*, (1989) and Henderson *et al.*, (1993).

In order to obtain quantitative data on the amount of pesticide absorbed by workers, it is necessary to understand the metabolism and pharmacokinetics of the compound in humans. This requirement has been dealt with in detail by Woollen (1993). Data from such human volunteer dosing studies enable a correct field sampling strategy and secondly define the body fluid matrix of choice. Ideally, this is urine as its collection is non-invasive and the collection of 24 hour voids is practicable. It is advisable to check the completeness of 24 hour urine collections by measuring the concentration of creatinine and expressing excretion as g/day. Substantially incomplete collections are readily apparent and can be either excluded or an allowance made (Woollen, 1993). Other parameters such as specific gravity and osmolarity may also be useful in this respect (Alessio *et al.*, 1985).

The need for metabolism and pharmacokinetic data is perceived by some as a major disadvantage of biological monitoring (NACA, 1985). However, this potential disadvantage must be judged in the light of the more accurate assessment of absorbed dose provided by a properly designed, interpretable biological monitoring study. This is the principal advantage of biological monitoring in the context of risk assessment for pesticides.

Some pesticides are unstable or highly volatile and therefore are not good candidates for ambient exposure monitoring, despite the efforts to accurately assess in field and storage and transit losses. Biological monitoring should be considered for such a pesticide and may be the only means of obtaining adequate quantitative data from which the absorbed dose can be derived.

If, for some technical or ethical consideration, a human volunteer study is regarded as impracticable, then animal metabolism and pharmacokinetic data may be taken into account. Primate studies have provided valuable information in this respect. It may be possible that if metabolism and excretion kinetics are similar in several animal species, then an assumption can be made that humans will metabolize and excrete the compound in a similar manner. However, there are clear examples which demonstrate the pitfalls when adopting this approach which are described in detail by Woollen (1993). Apart from interspecies differences in metabolism, there is the possibility of dose-dependent differences, pointing to the possible need for metabolism studies in animals and human volunteers at doses similar to the anticipated workplace exposures.

It is recommended that where a biological monitoring strategy is considered necessary for the pesticide in question, then urine is the preferred sampling matrix. Where possible and ethically feasible, metabolism and pharmacokinetic data derived from human volunteer studies should be considered as the optimum means of enabling an accurate estimate of the absorbed dose of the pesticide.

There is a need at the outset to consider the best sampling strategy for the compound in question. In particular, the toxicological profile of the compound must be evaluated in the context of its intended use patterns. The toxicity of the pesticide, the application equipment together with ambient dermal exposure data corrected for percutaneous absorption from an animal study, may militate against achieving an adequate margin of safety. Thus the greater precision provided by biological monitoring is needed.

Certain pesticides may not lend themselves to a biological monitoring strategy, for example if they are extensively metabolized to a large number of minor metabolites. A minor metabolite, particularly if subject to inter-individual variability in the proportion of the parent compound excreted as this moiety, does not provide an adequate basis for an accurate assessment of the absorbed dose of the compound. However, depending on the nature of the risk assessment, a minor metabolite can provide some useful information as a 'biological indicator' in the absence of more abundant biological monitoring markers.

## FIELD STORAGE AND STABILITY (RECOVERY) OF THE PESTICIDE

It is essential that the stability and recovery of the pesticide and its metabolites are determined from each of the relevant sampling matrices. It is recommended that, in general, field recovery determinations are made on each successive day of the study when exposure and absorbed dose are measured. Exceptions to making daily recovery assessments may be considered for compounds for which there are data from previous field studies demonstrating acceptable and consistent stability and recovery from the same matrices and under similar ambient conditions to those in the present study. In such cases, consideration should be given to reducing the number of occasions when field recovery samples are prepared.

Intersite variability within the same study should also be taken account of by preparing recovery samples at each site. If conditions are shown subsequently to be similar, it may not be necessary to analyse all the samples.

The area for field fortification work should be chosen carefully to avoid possible contamination with pesticide, for example from drift from the site of application.

## GENERAL FEATURES OF FIELD STUDY DESIGN

Before starting a study it should be considered whether ambient exposure and biological monitoring should be conducted concurrently in the field study. Both may be justified to provide data for inclusion in generic data bases, to examine the relationship between exposure and absorption and it also has the advantage of providing a second measurement should one fail. One useful feature of the tiered approach (Henderson, *et al.*, 1993) is that insight into the likely route(s) of exposure may be gained from the generic exposure databases, thus enabling a decision on which routes to concentrate on in the field study. For example, it is well established that mixing, loading and high volume application of non-volatile pesticides (other than wettable powder and dusty granular formulations) does not generate significant amounts of inspirable particulates. It therefore seems inappropriate to monitor inhalation exposure in such circumstances.

Other factors which may influence the choice of sampling strategy include possible concern over specific work activities during pesticide use. Exposure monitoring may be more useful in that it enables separate measurements of the respective contributions of these activities to the total exposure. However, if ambient exposure and biological monitoring are conducted concurrently then these contributions may be assessed simultaneously. Identification of the differences in the magnitude of exposure attributable to these activities permits the use of different regulatory options. An example is the recommended use of additional protective equipment during procedures with greater potential for exposure.

If adequate exposure data are available on the pesticide and use pattern in question, biological monitoring may be conducted on the subjects wearing their normal work clothing and any additional protective clothing and equipment as required by the label. This approach has the advantage of removing all doubt about possible interference of the exposure sampling dosimeters with the process of skin contamination and absorption.

As stated previously, the emphasis in this document is on maximum flexibility. This applies not only to the different approaches but also to the specific methodology used to determine the exposure or absorbed dose. For example, the investigator may believe that use of the dermal 'patch method' will provide adequate data for the purpose. It is essential that the necessary considerations for a scientifically sound protocol are followed and the approval of the regulatory authority sought.

An important consideration is that of the number of measurements of exposure and/or absorbed dose that are needed in the field study. This decision should be based on a consideration of the likely end-use of the data, the quality of the toxicological database, the nature of any identified toxicological endpoint, the required level of statistical confidence and the overall manageability of the field study. It is recommended that a sufficient number of measurements are made in different occupational settings which cover the range of use procedures and application equipment for which evaluation of exposure and/or absorbed dose is required. These comments also apply to crop re-entry procedures; for example, in harvesting, variation in work procedures may be substantial, even within the same crop.

The inherent variability in exposure under field conditions is best addressed by increasing the number of subjects, rather than repeated monitoring of the same individuals. Equally, consideration should be given to including as many sites as is feasible, rather than subjects using the same equipment under the same conditions. Certain types of pesticide application procedure render management of the study difficult, such as those involving aerial application. In such cases, repeated monitoring of the same individuals is a possible option. However, should biological monitoring be necessary a further limitation is introduced in that inter-individual variation in metabolism of the pesticide would be less well evaluated. The duration of the study will be prolonged owing to the possible need to collect urine samples over several days for each individual. The consequence of this is that repeat monitoring cannot commence until urine collection is complete. The use of biological monitoring in such circumstances should be considered only as a last resort.

Ideally, the duration of a replicate should be the whole working day, so that there is a greater chance that all the work activities which result in exposure, such as equipment repair and clean-up, are included. This point applies particularly to studies involving biological monitoring. Such data may not lend themselves to extrapolation on the basis of time or amount of active ingredient used in the same way as ambient exposure data.

The choice of use pattern (including application equipment) should be based on consideration of factors such as whether it is the predominant one for the product, or a minor one for which there are no generic data available to the investigator or regulatory authority to enable a risk assessment. The product should be used in the study at a representative recommended rate of application and on the likely maximum area of crop treatable in a working day under local conditions. It should also be applied in accordance with all the label recommendations for use. These principles also apply to studies involving crop re-entry and for which exposure should be determined after the shortest permissible re-entry period (if known).

Where the product label recommends the use of protective clothing and/or equipment, it is beneficial for such clothing and equipment to be provided to the workers by the supervisory team to ensure standardization. This will aid the scientific interpretation of the data, since the variable of differing standards of protection by different types of protective equipment will have been removed. Inclusion of criteria such as these ensure exposure and risk assessments for the product in accordance with the label recommendations. However, efforts should be made to ensure that the recommended protective clothing and equipment is practical and realistic.

There may be circumstances in which it is necessary to measure exposure under conditions of use which differ from those recommended, for example in post-registration surveillance of the pesticide in use. Examples of such circumstances include the availability of new toxicity data, the need to evaluate exposure for a new use pattern and the study of the possible influence of non or partial compliance with the label recommendations on the magnitude of exposure.

## TEST SUBJECTS

Normal agricultural workers (operators, workers or bystanders) should be the test subjects in a field study, rather than inexperienced volunteers. In cases where this is not possible, use of non-professional personnel may be considered, provided that they are given the requisite training in the handling and use of the pesticide and equipment. Males or females may be considered for inclusion in ambient exposure studies. However, in those studies involving biological monitoring, careful consideration must be given to the inclusion of both sexes in terms of impact on the interpretation of the metabolite excretion patterns owing to possible sex differences in metabolism and pharmacokinetics.

Informed consent of all subjects should be obtained by provision of the requisite information on the pesticide in an easily understood form. A form of consent should be signed by each subject. Test subjects should not be chosen on the basis of either known careful use of pesticides, or good personal hygiene and working practices; they should be representative of the working population under study. Furthermore, they should be told to use the pesticide and carry out work activities according to their normal practice. The subjects should consider themselves to be in normal good health. It is useful to give a simple questionnaire to the subjects before a field study to gather information about their experience in the use of pesticides and application equipment, their use of protective equipment and general health status. It should be made clear to all potential participants that they are free to withdraw from the monitoring study at any time. Consideration should be given to the provision of information to the subjects on their individual results.

## MANAGEMENT OF THE STUDY

The field study must be managed and supervised by people trained and experienced in the conduct of exposure studies. Emphasis should be placed upon training and evidence of competence of the supervisory team in the field sampling and observational procedures.

## QUALITY ASSURANCE

The field study should be conducted in accordance with the principles of Good Laboratory Practices as applied to field studies and recommended, for example, by the Organisation for Economic Co-operation and Development (1992) and others.

# GUIDELINES FOR THE CONDUCT OF FIELD STUDIES TO EVALUATE THE EXPOSURE OF OPERATORS, WORKERS AND BYSTANDERS TO PESTICIDES

## INTRODUCTION

Guidelines are proposed for the conduct of field studies to evaluate the exposure to, and absorption of, pesticides by operators, workers and bystanders during use and other agricultural activities. They are flexible in that the investigator can choose the most appropriate sampling methods in accordance with the tiered approach to exposure and risk assessment (Henderson *et al.*, 1993). If an investigator believes that some other methodology is better suited in the circumstances, and agreement in principle is obtained from the appropriate regulatory authority or other relevant organization then he should proceed. 'Standard Operating Procedures', although not included in these Guidelines, would be required to give the level of detail that is necessary for the successful conduct of a field exposure/biological monitoring study and to satisfy the requirements of Good Laboratory Practice (GLP) (e.g., OECD, 1992).

## PURPOSE OF GUIDELINES

The purpose of these Guidelines is to provide guidance on the measurement of the dermal and inhalation exposure to, and absorption of, pesticides by agricultural workers (operators, crop workers and bystanders). In certain circumstances the studies may fulfil a requirement to generate data for the European and other exposure databases such as the North American Pesticide Handlers Exposure Database and Predictive Operator Exposure Model, particularly for use patterns for which there are few if any data available. The study design therefore would have to take account of the primary requirements of the database.

## STUDY DESIGN

An appropriate number of test subjects is required for the study. The number of subjects involved will depend on the quality of the toxicity data for the pesticide as well as on the toxicological endpoint, the required degree of statistical validity and the overall manageability of the field study. As a general guide a minimum of 10 subjects is proposed. They should be located within easy travelling distance of each other to ensure ease of study management. Exposure to, and if necessary, the absorbed dose of, the pesticide should be measured during and following all work tasks involving potential contamination with the test material in a single day, at a representative label-recommended rate of application. Application should be to representative areas of crops. For activities such as crop harvesting, assessment should take place on the first day of permissible or possible re-entry.

Test subjects should be advised that all procedures, for example mixing, loading, application or harvesting, should be done in full compliance with the label precautions, particularly with regard to handling of the product with protective equipment and procedures for dealing with clean-up of spillage, cleaning out of equipment and repairs, and re-entry intervals. The precautions taken should not exceed those recommended on the label.

If assessment of absorption with biological monitoring is necessary, it is preferable that it be measured concurrently with exposure and the subjects should wear for example, standardized dermal exposure sampling clothing which is representative of what they would usually wear at this time of the year for application of pesticides. Exposure of the hands should be measured with for example, a handwash method whenever workers choose to wash their hands. For mixing and loading, clean up and repair procedures, protective equipment, consisting of for example, 'nitrile' protective gloves and vinyl faceshield, should be provided if recommended on the product label.

If only exposure is to be measured, then alternative methods may be used according to the investigator's preference. If considered appropriate, inhalation exposure should be measured using a personal air-sampling method. Airborne particulates in the inspirable range and/or vapour should be sampled in the breathing zone of each subject throughout his working day.

Any routine repair, clean-up and clean out procedures that are necessary during the day of assessment should be included in the measurement of exposure and absorption.

## LOCATION AND CROP

The locations for this study should be sites having the requisite minimum areas of the appropriate crop or treatment target. They should be selected on the basis of availability of typical loading and spray application equipment or work procedures such as crop harvesting. This choice will be made in conjunction with the selection of subjects willing to participate in the study. The exact locations of the sites should be known in advance.

Details should be recorded on total treatment area and the nature of the crop or treatment area, field sizes, harvested areas if appropriate and exact location. Field maps should be included in the Study File to enable future relocation of the trial site and reconstruction of the study if necessary.

## APPLICATION EQUIPMENT

Spray equipment should be that typically used for application of the product under study. If possible, a range of manufacturers' spray equipment should be included. Full technical details of the equipment should be recorded in the Study File and should include some or all of the following: tank capacity, filling method (open or closed, gravity or pump), pump type, presence of washing/rinsing facility, operating pressure, operating speed, boom length, boom line diameter, number of nozzles, type of nozzles, nozzle screen mesh size, type of nozzle check valve, open or closed cab, rate of application.

The spray application equipment should be checked by experienced personnel for correct operation and application rate before the start of work. Steps should be taken to ensure that the application rate is within acceptable limits. The application rate should be recorded.

Details of the application equipment and rate should be included in the Study File, together with any calibration data.

## FORMULATION AND PACKAGING

The formulation number and batch numbers if known should be recorded in the Study File.

The product should be supplied in typical and representative packaging. Full details of this packaging should be recorded in the Study File and should include size, orifice or neck diameter, design and nature of material from which it is manufactured.

The product may be supplied directly from a distributor. If at all possible, a sample of the product from the same production batch/lot should be obtained before the study to verify the specification. It is recognized however, that this may not be feasible in some circumstances. The certificate(s) of analysis should be obtained and included in the Study File.

## PROTECTIVE EQUIPMENT

If the product label specifies the use of protective clothing and/or equipment, (e.g., protective gloves and faceshield) it should be issued to the subjects before or on the morning of their day's use of the product, so that they may comply with the label precautions for its use.

## MEASUREMENT OF DERMAL EXPOSURE

The exposure sampling media (clothing or patches and gloves) should be donned by each subject or attached with assistance from a member of the supervisory team, before the start of his/her respective day's use of the test material and should be worn throughout the working day. This must include any clean-up and repair procedures that are necessary during the day and cleaning out of the equipment at the end of the day.

If the dosimeters should become wet with pesticide formulation or spray dilution to the point of saturation, they should be exchanged for fresh ones. These should be kept under close observation in case of further saturation.

Following removal, at a location free from contamination with the pesticide in question and with assistance from the study monitoring team where necessary, the sampling media should be prepared for storage.

If biological monitoring is to be conducted concurrently with exposure assessment, exposure of the hands may be measured by a handwash procedure which should be carried out whenever the subject wishes to wash his hands. This ensures that there is no interference with the process of dermal contamination and absorption. Aliquots of the handwash solution should be taken and prepared for storage.

If protective gloves are used during any procedures, they may also be taken for subsequent analysis of test material content together with any washings. Although these analytical data would not normally form part of the total exposure determinations, they may be useful in examining the relationship between the exposure of the hands (from the handwashes) and the contamination of the protective gloves.

All exposure samples should be stored temporarily in cool boxes containing dry ice or ice packs as necessary. They should be transferred to a deep-freeze as soon as possible. The times of sample collection and deposition in the deep-freeze should be recorded, as should all other essential sampling and storage information and included in the Study File.

## MEASUREMENT OF INHALATION EXPOSURE

The concentration of the test material as inspirable fraction may be measured in the breathing zone of each worker using personal air samplers and for example, closed-face cassettes containing suitable, analytically validated filters.

A sampling rate of 1 to 2 l/min is needed to provide an acceptable volume of air over the typical duration of a working day and may be a specific requirement for the type of sampler used. Flow rates should be calibrated both before and after sampling using a soap bubble meter or other suitable device such as a calibrated flowmeter. Details of flow rates, durations of sampling and total volumes of air sampled should be recorded and maintained in the Study File. Each air sampling pump should be checked intermittently throughout the working day to ensure its continued satisfactory operation.

On completion of sampling, filter cassettes should be stored temporarily in a cool box containing dry ice or ice packs as necessary. The samples should be transferred to the deep-freeze as soon as possible after collection.

Inhalation exposure samples should be stored in separate cool-boxes and freezer compartments to those used for dermal exposure, handwash and urine samples.

## MEASUREMENT OF ABSORBED (OR INTERNAL) DOSE (BIOLOGICAL MONITORING)

The subjects may be monitored for their excretion of an appropriate metabolite(s), (i.e., as identified preferably by a human volunteer metabolism study).

They should have had no recent exposure to the test material or similar pesticide prior to their day of use of the product. The exact exposure free period depends on the excretion kinetics of the compound determined preferably in humans. Twenty-four hour urine samples should be collected by subjects on the day before using the product (pre-exposure), the day of use and for each of several days afterwards (exact duration depending on the excretion kinetics). Collection of urine, using the containers provided, should start first thing in the morning and finish at approximately the same time the following morning. The first void of the day should be given in the container of the previous day's collection. For subsequent voids during the day, a fresh container should be used for the remainder of the 24 hour collection period. The containers should be available to the subjects at all times to ensure that all urine should be collected. The subjects must be instructed to exercise caution to ensure that contamination of the urine with test material during urination does not occur.

On completion of the day's work, the subjects should exercise normal hygiene practice in terms of washing or showering. They should have no subsequent contact with the test material or similar products for the total period of urine collection.

The one exception to this is if the application has to be carried over into a second day because of, for example, rainfall. If it is believed that exposure to other pesticides will not interfere with metabolism and analysis of the compound of interest, there is no reason why the subject should not continue to use unrelated pesticides, provided that a record is maintained of which ones and when they were used.

Each 24 hour sample should be measured for total volume and two sub-samples taken. These replicate samples will be stored separately in the deep-freeze. One set of samples (primary) may be shipped to the laboratory for analysis whilst the other set (reserve) remains in local, frozen storage as a reserve.

## FIELD STORAGE AND STABILITY (RECOVERY)

### Vehicle For Test Material

The objective of any field storage and stability study is to assess stability and recovery for the compound in the form in which it is present in the field. Therefore, for liquid formulations, the spray solution should be used for fortifying dermal and inhalation sampling matrices but only if it is uniformly mixed. On each day of measurement, a representative tank mix sample should be withdrawn from a spray nozzle, rather than the top of the spray tank, following the first mix-load of the day. This sample should be taken after sufficient time has elapsed to ensure homogeneity of the spray tank mixture after thorough agitation in the spray tank. This could not be guaranteed by withdrawing a sample from a spray tank immediately after mixing and loading.

For ready to use solid formulations and powders, consideration should be given to preparing pre-weighed aliquots in the laboratory and shipping them to the field for fortification purposes. In such cases, while recognizing the technical limitation, it is better to add the sampling matrix to the formulation in a vial rather than the converse to minimize potential loss of granules or powder.

An alternative to this procedure is to prepare and fortify with standard solutions of the test material, particularly if fortification at different concentrations is necessary. This does have the inherent disadvantage of the solution not being the physical form in which the test material is presented in the field. Stability and recovery in liquid and solid vehicles may be different.

### Fortification Levels

Consideration should be given to fortification of sampling matrices at different concentrations to cover the anticipated range of exposures. As a guide, the lowest concentration could be 10 times the limit of quantification. Prediction of the range of exposures may be assisted by reference to generic exposure databases. Fortification at different levels should be considered particularly for compounds known to be inherently unstable or volatile.

### Dermal Exposure Sampling Matrices

Four squares (approximately 25 $cm^2$) of each material should be fortified with spray solution at (3) concentrations. A set of 4 untreated controls for each material should also be included. Immediately after fortification two squares of each material, per fortification level, should be stored in a cool-box containing dry ice or ice packs as necessary. Two untreated control samples should be stored in the same manner.

To assess possible degradation under ambient conditions and exposure to light, two of the four squares per fortification level, together with a duplicate set of control samples, should be exposed to ambient conditions for a period of time equivalent to the duration of exposure (i.e., the working day). These exposed samples will be located on site but in a position free from contamination with, and drift of, test material.

Where two layers of sampling media are used to assess actual dermal exposure, recovery from both types of material, if different, should be assessed. Consideration should also be given to mimicking as closely as possible the study conditions in which one layer of sampling medium lies beneath the other one. This may be accomplished by placing squares of the outer sampling medium on top of fortified inner sampling medium squares.

Following exposure, at the end of the working day, the samples (treated and control) should be stored in a cool box containing dry ice or ice packs as necessary. All samples should be transferred to the deep-freeze as soon as possible after completion of the day's monitoring.

### Handwash/Handrinse

Stability and recovery of the test material from handwash solution or handrinse should be assessed at the same time as from the dermal exposure sampling matrices. Handwash solution may be freshly prepared by a member of the supervisory team on each day's use. This must be done at the outset before any possible contact with test material. The method of preparation should be as described previously for the measurement of hand exposure. Duplicate 200 ml aliquots of handwash or handrinse solution in suitable containers should be fortified with spray solution at (3) concentrations. A set of untreated controls should also be retained. Following fortification, samples should be stored in a cool-box containing dry ice or ice packs as necessary. At the end of the day, the samples should be transferred to the deep-freeze as soon as possible.

### Inhalation Exposure Sampling Matrices

Duplicate sets of filters (and/or adsorbent resin for vapour sampling, if appropriate) should be fortified by addition of aliquots of spray solution at (3) concentrations. A set of untreated control filters and absorbent resin tubes should also be prepared. Immediately following fortification each set should be taken and, where appropriate, connected to pre-calibrated air-sampling pumps in the same location as the dermal 'exposed' samples. These pumps should be operated at the same flow rate as the 'test' samples for a period of time approximately equivalent to the duration of sampling over the working day (it may not always be feasible to run the pumps if ambient air concentrations or contaminated dust concentrations of the pesticide in the area are high). On completion, the pump flow rate should be re-calibrated, the filter (and/or adsorbent resin tube) removed and stored in a cool box. The samples should be transferred to the deep-freeze as soon as possible.

### Urinary Metabolites

The stability of the metabolite(s) in stored urine should be assessed for each successive day of the study. Duplicate 50 ml urine samples from personnel unexposed to the test material should be fortified with metabolite(s) at (3) concentrations.

These fortified samples should be stored under the same ambient conditions as the test 24 hour samples from the workers for a similar period of time. Immediately after this period of ambient storage, the samples should be transferred in a cool box containing dry ice or ice packs to the deep-freeze. Primary samples should be separated from reserve samples which should remain in local storage until analysis of the primary set is complete. The standard solutions used for fortification should also be returned to the laboratory for checking of their concentrations, along with the primary set of samples.

### Sampling Of Spray Solutions Of Test Material

The samples of spray solution used for fortification of the dermal and inhalation exposure sampling matrices should be retained for checking of their concentration. They may be placed in the cool box immediately after fortification is complete. Owing to the possible problems with re-establishing homogeneity after thawing of spray solution samples, it is recommended that three aliquots are transferred to glass vials and placed directly in the deep-freeze. These samples may thus be analysed directly. Further, random samples of spray tank dilutions should be taken throughout the day's spraying as a check on concentration. Batch numbers and source of the product must be recorded.

## WEATHER CONDITIONS

Windspeed, direction, shade temperature and relative humidity should be monitored at frequent intervals at each site. Observations at approximately hourly intervals are recommended, or whenever significant changes are apparent.

The types of equipment used for such measurement should be recorded in the Study File. Where applicable they should have been calibrated before the study and the results of this calibration placed in the Study File.

## ADDITIONAL OBSERVATIONS

The amounts of test material used should be observed carefully and recorded. Detailed observation should be made of the loading and application equipment. Areas of crop, number and/or weight of crop commodities harvested should be recorded. Where appropriate the time between application of the pesticides and crop re-entry should be recorded. Work practices, particularly compliance with the label precautions, should be observed carefully and recorded. Photographic and video records of the study are recommended, where feasible.

## SHIPMENT OF SAMPLES

Following completion of the field phase of the study all samples should be shipped if necessary in a deep-frozen or cold condition to the laboratory for analysis. Due to the necessity for the samples to remain deep-frozen or cold, it is essential that proper, documented procedures are put in place to minimize the possibility of their thawing out or being lost in transit. The method and route of transport must therefore be known and arranged before shipment takes place. Appropriate 'chain of custody' documentation should be used to satisfy GLP needs in these respects.

## RESPONSIBILITIES OF THE STUDY (SUPERVISORY) TEAM

The responsibilities of each member of the team should be absolutely clear to him/her at the planning phase of the study. Each member should be given a copy of the protocol and all relevant 'Standard Operating Procedures'. Where necessary, training of team members should be undertaken by appropriately trained and experienced personnel, for example the Study Director or Principal Investigator. This should be done prior to the start of the study. Each team member should have a training record, signed by the approved 'trainer', to cover the aspects of the study with which they will be involved. If training records exist already, then they should be reviewed and, if necessary, updated. Copies of team members' training records should be included in the Study File, together with a list of their names.

## STUDY RECORDS

Standard forms may be used to document all parts of the field study, to cover:
Personal details of subjects, including relevant agricultural experience;
Trial location details, including site/field history and maps;
Details on number, size and design of formulation packs;
Details of application equipment;
Study team personnel;
Study data form, including loading, weather and sampling information;
Observations on work practice;
Calibration of air sampling pumps;
Spray tank sampling;
Records of urine volumes and dates of collection and sub-sampling;
Field fortification of dermal and inhalation exposure sampling matrices;
Field fortification or urinary metabolite(s);
Deep-freeze sample deposition;
'Chain of Custody' and other shipping information;
Incidents.

All the above documentation should be included in the Study File. Following completion of the field study all study records should be indexed and, following preparation of the final report, transferred to a GLP archive and stored for an indefinite period.

## EVALUATION OF EXPOSURE AND ABSORBED DOSE

The amounts of (test substance) on the dermal exposure sampling media permit an evaluation of the potential and actual dermal exposure of the subjects. The total potential exposure is the total amount of (test substance) recovered from all sampling clothing and handwashes.

The estimated actual exposure is derived from the amounts recovered from the inner sampling clothing, the handwashes or gloves if the subjects only wear one layer of clothing under the prevailing conditions.

An estimate of actual exposure may also be derived if subjects usually wear two layers of clothing. This is done by taking account of the outer to inner clothing transfer factor and correcting the amounts recovered from the inner clothing by this percent factor to estimate the contamination of the skin beneath plus the amounts recovered from the handwashes.

The units for expression of the exposure data in terms of (test substance) are:-

| | | |
|---|---|---|
| Dermal Exposure | : | mg/body part<br>mg/whole body/day<br>mg/kg bodyweight/day<br>mg/kg test material handled and/or applied |
| Inhalation Exposure | : | µg/m$^3$<br>µg/day *<br>µg/kg bodyweight/day<br>µg/kg test material handled and/or applied |
| Absorption | : | mg/day<br>mg/kg bodyweight/day |

* Calculated from duration of exposure and standardized ventilation rates according to level of work activity (U.S. EPA, 1986).

## REPORTING REQUIREMENTS

The following information is required:

1. Test material, purity, stability, product specification of formulation, batch numbers, nominal and actual concentrations;
2. Description of study design;
3. Exact locations of study sites;
4. Description of mixing, loading and application equipment, application rate(s) crop areas treated/harvested;
5. Description of work procedures of workers, to include any use of protective clothing and equipment;
6. Detailed description of all sampling methods used, e.g., dermal, inhalation, biological monitoring, environmental conditions, field recovery evaluation;
7. Conditions of sample storage and shipment;
8. Description of analytical methodology, extraction, detection, validation;
9. Calculations and extrapolation factors, e.g., breathing rates;
10. Results of analysis, to include uncorrected and corrected residues, laboratory and field recoveries, extrapolated exposure and absorbed dose values, environmental conditions;
11. Tabulation of:
    All relevant analytical data;
    Extrapolation results, e.g., dermal, inhalation, exposure, absorbed dose (from biological monitoring);
    Environmental conditions;
12. Photographic record;
13. Discussion and interpretation of results;
14. Conclusions;
15. Location of raw data;
16. References.

## REFERENCES


Abbott, I.M., Bonsall, J.L., Chester, G., Hart, T.B., and Turnbull, G.J., 1987, Worker exposure to a herbicide applied with ground sprayers in the United Kingdom, *Am. Ind. Hyg. Assoc. J.* 48:167-175.

Alessio, L., Bolin, A., Dell'Orto, A., Toffoletto, F., and Ghezzio, I., 1985, Reliability of urinary creatinine as a parameter used to adjust values of urinary biological indicators, *Int. Arch. Occup. Environ. Health* 55:99-106.

Berkow, S.G., 1931, Value of surface area proportions in the prognosis of cutaneous burns and scalds, *Amer. J. Surg.* 11:315-317.

Chester, G., Dick, J., Loftus, N.J., Woollen, B.H., and Anema, B.H., 1990, The effectiveness of protective gloves in reducing dermal exposure to, and absorption of, the herbicide fluazifop-P-butyl by mixer-loader-applicators using tractor sprayers, *7th. Int. Congr. of Pesticide Chemistry*, Vol III, p. 378, IUPAC.

Curry, P., and Iyengar, S., 1992, Comparison of exposure assessment guidelines for pesticides, *Rev. Environ. Contam. Toxicol.* 129:79-93.

Davis, J.E., 1980, Minimizing occupational exposure to pesticides: Personal monitoring, *Residue Rev.* 75:35-50.

Durham, W.F., and Wolfe, H.T., 1962, Measurement of the exposure of workers to pesticides, *Bull. WHO* 26:75-91.

Fenske, R.A., 1987, Assessment of dermal exposure to pesticides: a comparison of the patch technique and video-imaging/fluorescent tracer technique, *in:* Sixth International Congress on Pesticide Chemistry IUPAC, 579-82.

GIFAP, Groupement International des Associations Nationales de Fabricants de Produits Agrochemiques, 1990. Monitoring studies in the assessment of field worker exposure to pesticides. Technical Monograph No. 14, Bruxelles, Belgium.

Henderson, P.Th., Brouwer, D.H., Opdam, J.J.G., Stevenson, H., and Stouten, J.Th.J., 1993, Risk assessment for worker exposure to agricultural pesticides: Review of a workshop, *Ann. Occup. Hyg.* 37(5):499-507.
Lewis, R.G., 1976, Sampling and analysis of airborne pesticides in air pollution from pesticides and agricultural processes, R.E. Lee Jr., ed., CRC Press, Cleveland, Ohio.
Mull, R., and McCarthy, J.F., 1986, Guidelines for conducting mixer-loader-applicator studies, *Vet. Hum. Toxicol.* 28(4):328-336.
NACA, National Agricultural Chemicals Association, 1985, Guidelines for Conducting Biological Monitoring - Applicator Exposure Studies, NACA, Washington, D.C.
Organisation for Economic Co-operation and Development, 1992, GLP Consensus Document. The Application of the GLP Principles to Field Studies, Environment Monograph No. 50, OECD Series on Principles of Good Laboratory Practice and Compliance Monitoring No. 6.
Peoples, S.A., and Knaak, J., 1982, Monitoring pesticide blood cholinesterase and analysing blood and urine for pesticides and their metabolites in pesticide residues and exposure, *in:* ACS Symp. Series No. 182:41-57, J.R. Plimmer, ed., American Chemical Society, Washington, D.C.
PHED, 1992, Pesticide Handlers Exposure Database. United States Environmental Protection Agency, Health and Welfare Canada, National Agricultural Chemicals Association.
Popendorf, W.J., and Leffingwell, J.T., 1982, Regulating organophosphate pesticide residues for farmworker protection, *Residue Rev.* 82:125-201.
Thongsinthusak, T., Ross, J.H., and Meinders, D., 1993, Guidance for the preparation of human pesticide exposure documents, HS-1612, May 4, California Environmental Protection Agency, Worker Health and Safety Branch.
U.S. Environmental Protection Agency, 1986, Pesticide Assessment Guidelines, Subdivision U, Applicator Exposure Monitoring, U.S. EPA, Washington, D.C.
Van Dyk, L.P., and Visweswariah, K., 1975, Pesticides in air: Sampling methods, *Residue Rev.* 55:91-134.
Van Heemstra-Lequin, E.A.H., and Van Sittert, N.J., eds, 1986, Biological monitoring of workers manufacturing, formulating and applying pesticides, *Tox. Lett.* 33:1-236, Elsevier, Amsterdam.
Vincent, J.H., and Mark, D., 1987, Comparison of criteria for defining inspirable aerosol and the development of appropriate samplers, *Am. Ind. Hyg. Assoc. J.* 48:451-457.
Wang, R.G.M., Franklin, C.A., Honeycutt, R.C., and Reinert, J.C., 1989, "Biological Monitoring for Pesticide Exposure: Measurement, Estimation and Risk Reduction", ACS Symp. Series No. 382, American Chemical Society, Washington, D.C.
Wolfe, H.R., 1976, Field exposure to airborne pesticides, *in:* Air Pollution from Pesticides and Agricultural Processes, R.E. Lee, Jr., ed., CRC Press, Cleveland, Ohio.
Woollen, B.H., 1993, Biological monitoring for pesticide absorption, *Ann. Occup. Hyg.* 37(5):525-540.
World Health Organization, 1975, Survey of exposure to organophosphorus pesticides in agriculture. Standard Protocol, VBC/75.9, WHO, Geneva.
World Health Organization, 1982, Field surveys of exposure to pesticides. Standard Protocol, VBC/82.1, WHO, Geneva.

# STUDY DESIGN CONSIDERATIONS FOR OCCUPATIONAL PESTICIDE EXPOSURE ASSESSMENT

Richard A. Fenske[1] and Kay Teschke[2]

[1]Department of Environmental Health, SC-34
School of Public Health and Community Medicine
University of Washington, Seattle WA 98195

[2]Department of Health Care and Epidemiology
University of British Columbia
Vancouver, British Columbia V6T 1Z3

## INTRODUCTION

Exposure assessments in occupational hygiene are normally conducted for one of four purposes: 1) hazard evaluation leading to appropriate control efforts, 2) monitoring to ensure compliance with workplace standards, 3) dose-response characterization within the context of epidemiological studies, and 4) estimation of dose or uptake for risk assessments. Assessment strategies and measurement techniques will differ depending on the purpose at hand. The Guidance Document[1] prepared for the Ottawa *Workshop on Methods of Pesticide Exposure Assessment* has been developed within the context of risk assessment. The goal of the Document is to establish an "internationally accepted, harmonized approach" to pesticide exposure assessment by providing pesticide registrants with guidelines for conducting exposure assessment studies which can be submitted to regulatory agencies in support of the registration or reregistration of specific agricultural chemicals. The Guidance Document reflects substantial progress in our understanding of pesticide exposure processes, and is intended to supersede previous guidance documents in this field.[2-4]

Studies required by regulatory agencies for the purpose of risk assessment have been referred to as "mandated science",[5] and can be distinguished from exploratory or hypothesis-driven science by their need to produce data which can withstand detailed regulatory review and quite possibly legal challenges. Normally such studies are limited in their design and methods to adhere to conventionally accepted procedures; indeed, this Workshop itself is an exercise in mandated science, with a primary goal of building scientific consensus regarding standard exposure assessment procedures. In this context the Guidance Document is exceptional in that it proposes novel approaches to pesticide exposure evaluation; in particular, its emphasis on field biomonitoring in conjunction with laboratory-based human pharmacokinetic studies represents a major advance in this field.

The Guidance Document is part of a broader risk management strategy in the field of pesticide exposure assessment which includes use of existing data and modelling techniques within a decision matrix or tier approach.[6] The tier approach proposes to employ generic exposure databases recently developed in North America and Europe in combination with assumptions and experimentally-derived standard factors to generate surrogate exposure estimates for pesticide registration. A comprehensive review of the benefits and pitfalls of the use of such databases was published recently by van Hemmen.[7] It is most important to recognize that measurements in existing exposure databases were collected under study designs which often placed constraints on exposure variability, as discussed below, and that these data are therefore of limited value in estimating current exposures. The proposal by van Hemmen to consider the 90th percentile of these data as the most appropriate estimate of exposure is well-grounded and should be endorsed by this Workshop.

## OCCUPATIONAL HYGIENE EXPOSURE ASSESSMENT STRATEGIES

Current risk assessment procedures require knowledge of the population at risk and the distribution of exposures within this population, as well as information on the toxicity of the compound under evaluation.[8] The primary goal of an exposure assessment strategy conducted in support of risk assessment is to identify a study population which is representative of the population at risk, and to then conduct a sampling program which characterizes well the central tendency and variability of the exposures which these individuals receive. In support of this goal four fundamental study design concerns can be reviewed briefly: the development of standard practices in exposure assessment, the stratification of workers into subpopulations for sampling, the selection of an appropriate sampling strategy, and the use of appropriate statistical analysis.

### Good Exposure Assessment Practices

Hawkins *et al.*,[9] recently proposed a rationale and framework for the conduct of exposure assessments in support of risk management decisions, and outlined eight "good exposure assessment practices" (GEAP), essentially an extension of Good Laboratory Practices (GLP) to field studies. In fact pesticide exposure assessment studies have long recognized the need for rigorous field GLP procedures. Thus it is not surprising that for five of the proposed GEAP — Protocol, Organization, Quality Assurance, Archiving, Communication of Results — the Guidance Document meets or exceeds the expectations of these authors. The remaining practices — Study Model, Study Design and Statement of Overall Uncertainty — are addressed only generally by the Guidance Document, and would need to be specified prior to initiation of a study. A discussion of statistical concepts which underlay these practices is presented at a later point in this review.

### Worker Stratification

Occupational hygienists have traditionally evaluated exposures according to job title or work activity within industrial settings.[10] Grouping workers in these ways tends to increase the precision of estimated mean exposures. One recent example of a worker grouping is the homogeneous exposure group, which has been proposed as a basis for reducing sampling burden for making compliance decisions.[11] Assignment of workers to such groups can presumably be done *a priori* through knowledge of environmental conditions and time-activity patterns, although Kromhout and colleagues have demonstrated that such classifications are not necessarily accurate.[12] In the case of agricultural worker exposure researchers have subdivided worker populations into such categories as pesticide handlers or fieldworkers, recognizing that exposure processes are markedly different for these groups. The categorization of workers by van Hemmen according to work activity, environment and application techniques represents the most thorough analysis to date of exposure variability within and across mixer/loader and applicator groups.[7] Krieger and colleagues have provided a similar analysis for agricultural field workers.[13] Furthermore, regulatory agencies require exposure data that are specific to crops and work activities in order to determine use restrictions, protective clothing requirements and other control strategies. Thus, the stratification of pesticide-exposed workers for exposure evaluation is a process dictated primarily by practical rather than statistical considerations.

## Sampling Strategy Selection

Once appropriate subpopulations of agricultural workers have been defined, the question remains as to how these groups should be sampled. The fundamental issues in field study design can be outlined by a series of simple interrogatives: who, where, when, how long, how often, how many?[14-15] The answers to these questions require substantial prior knowledge of worker populations and working conditions, as well as the toxicological and metabolic characteristics of the pesticide. An optimal field study protocol would be constructed of an idealized study design tempered by the practical difficulties inherent in human population studies as well as financial limitations.

An extremely important consideration in sampling strategy selection is recognition that for air sampling in industrial settings exposure variability is usually much greater than measurement (analytical) variability.[16] Consider for a moment the relative expense of data samples and quality assurance samples under a study scenario outlined in the Guidance Document. Table 1 indicates that if four different garments were used as sampling devices, then a total of 100 quality assurance samples would be collected per workday/site in contrast to only 12 data samples. Thus, quality assurance samples would represent about 90% of the total analytical load. The number of quality assurance samples could be reduced if a number of workers were sampled at the same site on the same day, or if a single type of dermal sampling garment was used, but the samples aimed at documenting analytical variability would remain a substantial proportion of total samples. The danger in this imbalance is that stringent quality assurance requirements may limit severely the sample sizes of study populations, and thus the ability of the study to adequately characterize exposure variability.

Virtually all pesticide exposure assessment studies conducted under current guidelines employ a "quasi-experimental" sampling strategy; i.e., a group of workers are recruited for the study and asked to conduct a single episode of pesticide handling with some constraints placed on exposure variability. The Guidance Document does not alter substantially this fundamental approach. Teschke *et al.*[17-18] examined available strategies for assessing fungicide exposure in the lumber industry, and concluded that representative sampling would provide the most accurate assessment of current exposures, in contrast to modelling, use of existing data or quasi-experimental approaches. The rationale for rejecting the use of quasi-experimental studies in this industry was three-fold: 1) such studies were unlikely to represent the full range of conditions which influence exposure; 2) this approach did not allow enumeration of the exposed population; and 3) small numbers of measurements collected under the constraints of quasi-experimental studies were likely to introduce bias into the exposure assessment. These issues are pertinent to the role of study design under review here, and are discussed in the following section.

**Table 1.** Comparison of Exposure Samples and Quality Assurance Samples Collected for One Workshift under Guidance Document Procedures

| SAMPLE TYPE | EXPOSURE SAMPLES Collection | Analysis | QUALITY ASSURANCE SAMPLES |
|---|---|---|---|
| DERMAL EXPOSURE[a] | | | |
| T-shirt | 1[b] | 1 | 16 |
| Long-sleeved shirt | 1 | 1 | 16 |
| Socks | 1 | 1 | 16 |
| Trousers | 1 | 1 | 16 |
| Handwash | 5[c] | 2[f] | 8 |
| INHALATION EXPOSURE | | | |
| Filters | 2[d] | 1[g] | 8 |
| Absorbent | 2 | 1 | 8 |
| BIOMONITORING | 4[e] | 4 | 6 |
| SPRAY SOLUTION | | | |
| Fortification solution | --- | --- | 3 |
| Random samples | --- | --- | 3 |
| TOTAL SAMPLES | 17 | 12 | 100 |

[a]Uses refined whole body method described in Guidance Document; assumes materials for garments are different.
[b]Assumes worker wears same clothes all day.
[c]Assumes washing prewash, mid-a.m., noon, mid-p.m. and p.m.
[d]Assumes change of media at noon.
[e]Assumes one 24 hr. pre- and three 24 hr. post-exposure collections.
[f]Assumes four handwashes are pooled (+ one pre-wash).
[g]Pre-wash + all other samples pooled.

One means of overcoming the criticisms of the quasi-experimental design is to conduct studies aimed at the most highly exposed portion of a population, the so-called "worst case" design. It can be argued that this approach is cost-efficient, since a single study of this kind may indicate no significant risk, thereby obviating the need for additional studies. In practice, however, the creation of a truly worst-case scenario is complicated and may be considered unethical. Furthermore, it may be difficult to determine *a priori* the most highly exposed groups or most hazardous working conditions, as mentioned previously. Finally, such studies provide very little information on actual exposure levels among the population at risk.

## Statistical Analysis

The role of statistical principles in study design has been the subject of extensive discussion within the occupational hygiene community.[11,18-19] Analysis of occupational hygiene air sampling data has led to the generalization that occupational exposures are log-normally distributed, both within and between workers.[19] Analysis of data sets generated by the North American Pesticide Handlers Exposure Database (PHED) indicates similar distribution patterns.[20] It has been concluded by most researchers in this field that the arithmetic mean exposure is the most appropriate statistic to summarize the central tendency of these types of exposure distributions for individual workers (within-worker), because of the direct relationship to cumulative dose under chronic low level exposure conditions.[11,19] However, the geometric mean exposure of a stratum of workers (between-worker) is the most logical basis from which to calculate exposure percentiles within the group; e.g., 95th, 90th, 50th percentiles.[18] The variance in exposure for both individual workers and groups of workers is best described by the geometric standard deviation. Hawkins and colleagues[11] have indicated that 6-11 samples may be sufficient to estimate mean exposures, but that larger sample sizes (20 or more) are needed to estimate reliably the variance. Buringh and Lanting[21] have conducted exposure modelling exercises and have also concluded that exposure variance will likely be underestimated if too few samples are taken. In situations where only a few samples can be taken, a conservative (i.e., high) estimate of the variance can be employed. Clearly the application of statistical principles to study design is an important issue deserving of far greater attention within the pesticide exposure assessment community.

## STUDY DESIGN FACTORS AFFECTING EXPOSURE VARIABILITY

All measurements of exposure will exhibit variability due to imprecision in sampling techniques or analytical procedures, and more importantly due to the exposure conditions and the natural behaviour of the subject of study. If variability is random then the central tendency of the exposure distribution will represent true exposure and the variance will provide an estimate of the certainty of the exposure value. If, however, some characteristic of the procedure causes measured exposure values to be skewed systematically then the true value will not be accurately reflected in the central tendency of the data. Such an effect is referred to as *bias* in epidemiology and occupational hygiene.[22]

The United States Environmental Protection Agency published guidelines for conducting exposure assessments in 1987.[2] It is largely on the basis of this document, and its precursor,[23] that generic exposure data have been collected and submitted to the North American Pesticide Handlers Exposure Database (PHED).[20] These guidelines can be criticized for their failure to recognize that certain practices may lead to bias in the exposure measurements generated. Sources of potential bias in pesticide exposure assessments will be discussed here in three categories: those for which the Guidance Document represents an advance in study design, those which place constraints on exposure variability, and those which remain in need of clarification.

### Study Design Advances

**Population Selection.** The Guidance Document argues that study participants should have substantial experience with the activity under study and that they should use their own equipment on their own property (i.e., "normal agricultural workers"). This explicit language is a marked improvement over the ambiguous guidance found in Subdivision U, and this approach should lead to a more representative sample of exposures. The Guidance Document also indicates that a single individual should not be used repeatedly as a subject (i.e., "increased number of subjects rather than repeated monitoring of same individuals"). The practice of using one individual to produce a large number of "replicates", tolerated under EPA guidelines, clearly has the effect of artificially reducing between-worker variability in the exposure data. Most workplace exposure studies indicate that total variability is greater than within-worker variability.[12,19]

**Duration of Measurements.** The document calls for full workshift sampling, the norm in occupational hygiene. Since the primary aim of these studies is to determine risks associated with chronic exposures, full workshift samples are required to represent true daily exposures. In cases where acute toxicity is of primary concern shorter sampling periods may be appropriate. Again this is a marked improvement over Subdivision U, which requires only that exterior sampling material have measurable levels of residues, resulting in some cases in samples of 10-20 minutes in duration.

**Application Conditions.** The Guidance Document proposes that the "product be used at a representative recommended rate of application" on "likely maximum area of crop". Regulatory agencies currently call for applications at maximum label rate, thus introducing a worst case or upper bound condition into the study design. The use of representative rates will result in a more accurate estimate exposure, but this benefit should be weighed against the need for regulatory agencies to ensure that legal use of the compound will not result in unacceptable exposures.

**Study Design Constraints on Exposure Variability**

**Label Compliance Constraints.** The document states that "test subjects should be advised that all procedures should be done in full compliance with the label precautions"; and that "precautions should not exceed those recommended on the label". These requirements ensure that behaviours prohibited by the label will not occur, with a likely reduction in true exposure values and their variability.

**Protective Clothing Constraints.** The Document states that protective clothing "should be provided if recommended on the product label"; and that it "should be issued to the subjects before or on the morning of their day's use of the product, so that they may comply with the label precautions for its use". The consistent use of new chemical protective clothing (CPC) cannot be considered a normal practice among the exposed populations at this time. This requirement is very likely to reduce exposures, since much dermal exposure is believed to result from inconsistent use, contamination and deterioration of CPC.

**Equipment Constraints.** The Document states that "the spray application equipment should be checked by experienced personnel for correct operation and application rate before the start of work. Steps should be taken to ensure that the application rate is within acceptable limits". These actions are likely to eliminate or greatly reduce the incidence of accidents, mechanical repairs, and inadvertent over-applications due to miscalibration, resulting in reduced exposures compared to normal agricultural practices.

**Study Design Issues to be Addressed**

**Sampling Locations.** The Document provides very little guidance in regard to site selection, stating only that sampling should occur at "as many sites as feasible". There is clearly a need here to develop selection criteria for sites, and to ensure that these sites will be representative of sites of concern.

**Seasonal Effects.** No guidance regarding when to sample is provided. One notable effect of season is the proper use of protective clothing. In many parts of the

United States, for example, compliance with label requirements may occur in the spring, fall or winter, but not during the hotter months of summer. The effect of season on exposure has been documented in the timber mill industry, and it has been recommended that studies incorporate a seasonal component into their designs.[18]

**Sample Size.** The Guidance Document indicates that sample size should be based on the quality and nature of toxicological information and practical concerns related to the manageability of the field study, and recommends as a general guide a minimum of 10 measurements. Teschke and colleagues have argued that a random sample of ten is sufficient to calculate a mean exposure value, but that the variance derived from such a sample cannot be considered reliable. They concluded that for sample sizes less than 30 a conservative estimate of the variance should be employed in determining percentile distributions from exposure data.[18]

**Observational Bias.** The Document proposes that in most cases workers be studied for one day, although biological monitoring may continue beyond the study day. This approach has been referred to as a single exposure design,[24] and has been used widely in recent assessment studies. However, workers' initial involvement in a study is a time when they are acutely aware that their performance is under scrutiny. Thus, behaviour on the first day of the study is not likely to be typical. Nigg (personal communication) has noted significant behavioral changes among subjects on subsequent study days, with differences evident in their exposure values. No current or proposed guidelines have addressed this issue, although it is common practice in many other human population studies to design procedures to control for this effect.

**Motivational Bias.** What leads some workers to join pesticide exposure assessment studies when others do not? Since current human subjects guidelines require that participation in such studies must be voluntary, self-selection is a primary factor defining study populations. Several concerns can be raised here. First, financial incentives may be required to induce participation, particularly in studies which require complete urine collection on multiple days. Yet workers who are paid for their participation may feel the need to perform well; i.e., to conduct applications in a careful manner. Second, those workers who routinely practice good health and safety may be much more willing to participate than those who feel that their normal behaviour will be viewed critically. Third, in some cases a product undergoing registration review is perceived as highly beneficial among users. If so, they may develop "loyalty" to the product, and be inclined to do the best they can to see that it garners approval. These concerns should be viewed as speculative since no data are available to support them, but it appears prudent to consider that subject motivation can exert influence on exposure values.

## Post-Registration Study Design

Pesticide exposure assessment should not end with registration. Once a compound has come into general use, effective product stewardship should include periodic sampling of the exposed population and review of these data by regulatory agencies. Given the wide variety of equipment, application procedures, and work practices, it is essential to determine whether in fact the exposure estimates derived from a combination of database information, assumptions, standard factors and controlled exposure trials reflect true exposure distributions in the exposed populations.[5] Risk management decisions based on risk assessments, margins of uncertainty, and feasibility considerations represent predictions that adverse health effects will not occur in the exposed population. Follow-up studies would ensure that these predictions were indeed accurate, and would provide a scientific foundation for altering regulations and conducting epidemiological research.

The key design components of such post-registration studies have been outlined previously.[18] They are 1) enumeration of the exposed population, 2) stratification by worker group, 3) random sampling within each strata, and 4) calculation of the mean and variance of exposure within each group such that exposure distribution percentiles can be determined. If sample sizes were small in such studies, it would be necessary to employ conservative estimates of the variance.

The Guidance Document represents a major step forward in the field of pesticide exposure assessment, and provides a sound methodological foundation for determining exposures associated with the use of these compounds. Integration of the study design considerations discussed here will further strengthen the scientific validity of field investigations. Data generated by these guidelines will be instrumental in setting safe standards for occupational exposures to pesticides.

## REFERENCES


1. Chester, G., Guidance document: The conduct of field studies to evaluate the exposure of operators, workers and bystanders to pesticides, *in:* Proceedings of the Workshop on Methods of Pesticide Exposure Assessment, October 5-8, 1993, Ottawa, (1995).
2. U.S. Environmental Protection Agency. Pesticide Assessment Guidelines, Subdivision U, Applicator Exposure Monitoring, U.S. Department of Commerce National Technical Information Service, Washington, D.C. (1986).
3. U.S. Environmental Protection Agency. Pesticide Assessment Guidelines, Subdivision K, Exposure: Reentry Protection, U.S. Department of Commerce National Technical Information Service, Washington, D.C. (1986).
4. World Health Organization. Field surveys of exposure to pesticides standard protocol, *Toxicol. Lett.* 3:223-235 (1986).
5. Salter, L., Mandated Science: Science and Scientists in the Making of Standards, Kluwer Academic Publishers, London (1988).
6. Carmichael, N.G., Pesticide exposure: Overview of the tier approach, *in:* Proceedings of the Workshop on Methods of Pesticide Exposure Assessment, October 5-8, 1993, Ottawa, (1995).
7. Van Hemmen, J.J., Agricultural pesticide exposure data bases for risk assessment, *Rev. Environ. Contam. Toxicol.* 126:1-85 (1992).
8. National Academy of Sciences. Risk Assessment in the Federal Government: Managing the Process, National Academy Press, Washington, D.C.
9. Hawkins, N.C., Jayjock, M.A., and Lynch, J., A rationale and framework for establishing the quality of human exposure assessments, *Am. Ind. Hyg. Assoc. J.* 53(1):34-41.
10. Corn, M., and Esmen, N.A., Workplace exposure zones for classification of employee exposures to physical and chemical agents, *Am. Ind. Hyg. Assoc. J.* 40:47-57 (1979).
11. Hawkins, N.C., Norwood, S.K., and Rock, J.C., A Strategy for Occupational Exposure Assessment, American Industrial Hygiene Association, Akron, OH (1991).
12. Kromhout, H., Symanski, E., and Rappaport, S.M., A comprehensive evaluation of within and between worker components of occupational exposure to chemical agents, *Ann. Occ. Hyg.* 37:253-270 (1993).
13. Krieger, R.I., Ross, J.H., and Thongsinthusak, T., Assessing human exposure to pesticides, *Rev. Environ. Contam. Toxicol.* 128:1-69 (1992).
14. Roach, S.A., A more rational basis for air-sampling programs, *Am. Ind. Hyg. Assoc. J.* 27:1-12 (1966).
15. Corn, M., Strategies of air sampling, *Scand. J. Work Environ. Health.* 11:173-80 (1985).
16. Nicas, M., Simmons, B.P., and Spear, R.C., Environmental versus analytical variability in exposure measurements, *Am. Ind. Hyg. Assoc. J.* 52(12):553-7 (1991).
17. Teschke, K., Marion, S.A., Jin, A., Fenske, R.A., and Van Netten, C., Strategies for determining occupational exposures in risk assessments: A review and a proposal for assessing fungicide exposures in the lumber industry, *Am. Ind. Hyg. Assoc. J.* 55:443-449 (1994).

18. Teschke, K., Fenske, R.A., Van Netten, C., Jin, A., and Marion, S.A. Generic Guidelines for Assessing Worker Exposure to Antisapstain Chemicals in the Lumber Industry, Report to the Health Monitoring Sub-Committee of the B.C. Stakeholder Forum on Sapstain Control. Vancouver, University of British Columbia (report available from the authors) (1992).
19. Rappaport, S.M., Assessment of long-term exposures to toxic substances in air, *Ann. Occup. Hyg.* 35:61-121 (1991).
20. Pesticide Handler Exposure Database (PHED). VERSAR, Inc., Arlington, VA (1992).
21. Buringh, E., and Lanting, R., Exposure variability in the workplace: Its implications for the assessment of compliance, *Am. Ind. Hyg. Assoc. J.* 52:6-13 (1991).
22. Checkoway, H., Pearce, N.E., and Crawford-Brown, D.G., Research Methods in Occupational Epidemiology, Oxford University Press, New York.
23. Davis, J.E., Minimizing occupational exposure to pesticides: Personnel monitoring, *Residue Rev.* 75:33-50 (1980).
24. Fenske, R.A., Validation of environmental monitoring by biological monitoring: the fluorescent tacer technique and the patch technique, *in:* Biological Monitoring for Pesticide Exposure, R.A. Wang et al., eds., ACS Symp. Series 382:70-84, American Chemical Society, Washington DC (1989).

# GUIDANCE DOCUMENT: QUALITY ASSURANCE / QUALITY CONTROL

Curt Lunchick

Jellinek, Schwartz & Connolly, Inc.
Arlington, VA 22209

The quality control aspects of pesticide exposure field studies are critical to the acceptability of a study to regulating agencies, yet it often remains as the least planned portion of the study. The EPA's Occupational and Residential Exposure Branch has determined that a large plurality of the exposure studies that they reject, were rejected on the basis of inadequate quality control data. To reduce the rejection of studies based on QA/QC, the guidance document should contain a separate section clearly delineating the QA/QC requirements in explicit detail.

Subdivision U of EPA's Pesticide Assessment Guidelines deals with applicator exposure monitoring and discusses the quality control aspects of the field studies in reasonably good detail. However, the discussion of QC is interspersed with monitoring methodology discussions and the impact on the importance of QC is lost to the reader. The guidance document we are discussing at the workshop should have a separate detailed section devoted to the quality control aspects of the study. The purpose of this QC section is to guide the reader to understanding exactly what is expected to support the quality control of the exposure study.

The quality control section of the guidance document should provide the reader with step-by-step guidance on what quality control data are necessary to support the field exposure study data. I would suggest the following subsections.

1. Definitions
2. Analytical Method Development and Validation
3. Fortification Levels
4. Pre-study Laboratory Recoveries
5. Storage Stability
6. Pre-Study Field Recoveries
7. Field Quality Control Sampling
    a. Field controls (blanks)
    b. Field Recoveries
    c. Tank mix sampling

*Methods of Pesticide Exposure Assessment*, Edited by
P.B. Curry *et al.*, Plenum Press, New York, 1995

8. Laboratory Sample Analysis Quality Control
    a. Concurrent Laboratory recovery with each sample run
9. Adjustment of data based on Quality Control Analysis

As stated previously, the purpose of each section would be to provide the user of the guidance document with the necessary guidance to develop a study with the appropriate quality control data to support the acceptance of the exposure data by the regulatory agencies.

A definitions section is important to standardize terminology. This guidance document is intended for international reference and standardizing terminology is vital to minimize misunderstanding.

I have reviewed the guidance for conducting study quality control recommended by Graham Chester in the guidance document and I have also reviewed the working draft of "QC/QA and Study Design Proposals For Worker Exposure Studies" prepared by Monty Eberhart and Ed Dow, for review by EPA. Merging the recommendations provided in both documents will provide the detailed guidance necessary to permit the guideline document to fulfill its purpose.

I am not going to go into a detailed discussion on the recommendations concerning the number of samples recommended for the acceptable criteria for recoveries and variability. I strongly believe; however, that three analyzed samples per matrix and fortification level should be a minimum requirement. Additional samples can be taken and stored in reserve.

I would like to raise several topics for discussion. The use and analysis of the spray tank solution is a topic that I believe requires further discussion. Graham suggests that for liquid formulations, the spray solution should be used for fortifying dermal and inhalation sampling matrices, if the formulation is uniformly mixed. To avoid the heterogenicity of formulation dispersal in the spray tank, sampling from a spray nozzle is recommended. I agree that sampling from the nozzle should provide a more representative sample than a sample removed from the spray tank. One caution is the possible risk to the sampler if the pesticide is very acutely toxic.

Field fortification with the spray solution makes sense if the spray solution is analyzed for actual concentration of active ingredient. Assuming the nominal concentration for the spray solution would be unacceptable and lead to errors in the calculation of field recoveries. This is because measured spray tank concentrations of the active ingredient can be substantially different from the intended concentrations.

The variation in spray tank solution concentrations also raises another quality control issue. Should the nominal quantity of pesticide sprayed be adjusted based on the analytical quantification of spray solution concentration? Generally when exposure is calculated on a mg/kg a.i. basis, the kg of active ingredient is based on what we assume the mixer/loader put into the spray tank. Yet what assurance do we have that the proper quantity of pesticide was mixed? Investigators who have sampled the spray tank solution frequently obtain concentrations quite different from what is expected. Is this from lack of spray tank homogenicity or mixing error? An extra liter of a 4EC product in the spray tank means an extra half kilo of active ingredient. Therefore, if the spray solution analysis indicates that the concentration was 120% of nominal or 60% of nominal, should the amount of active ingredient we assume was sprayed be adjusted accordingly? The guidance document recommends sampling of spray solutions. I support that, but only if we know what to do with the results.

One final area that I would like to hear discussions on concerns the field spike procedures for formulations applied as a solid. I would discourage the use of the technical grade formulation or the solid formulation dissolved in a solvent as the field spike solution. Neither procedure necessarily represents the fate in the field of the active ingredient in the solid formulation. Adjusting the field samples of a solid formulation by the field recovery of the technical grade active ingredient of a solvent dissolved derivative is probably as accurate as selecting the field recovery from a random numbers table. I do believe that the guidance document's suggestion of using pre-weighed aliquots of the solid formulations has merit. I would like to see a more detailed discussion of the procedure in the guidance document.

GUIDANCE DOCUMENT

# A CRITIQUE OF PHARMACOKINETICS AND BIOLOGICAL MONITORING

Delmont C. Eberhart

MILES Inc.
Agriculture Division
Product Safety Section
Research and Development Department
Kansas City, Missouri 64120

## INTRODUCTION

The purpose of this discussion is to critique the OECD Guidance Document entitled: "The Conduct of Field Studies to Evaluate the Exposure of Operators, Workers and Bystanders to Pesticides" with respect to pharmacokinetics and biological monitoring.

I would like to begin by acknowledging the significant efforts of our colleagues, Graham Chester and Bruce Woollen of Zeneca Agrochemicals, in promoting the development of biological monitoring as a quantitative exposure assessment technique for pesticides. Most of us have recognized for some time that biological monitoring represents an important next step in our understanding of pesticide exposures and risk assessment. For a number of reasons, however, the amount of work dedicated to this approach has been less than might be expected based on its potential to provide more accurate exposure data for risk assessment and risk management decisions. I believe that the recent work of Chester (Chester, 1993; Chester, *et al.*, 1987; Chester and Hart, 1986) Woollen (Woollen, 1993; Woollen, *et al.*, 1992; Woollen, *et al.*, 1991) and others (Ramsey, *et al.*, 1992; Carmichael, *et al.*, 1989; Dubelman and Cowell, 1989; Nolan, *et al.*, 1984) provides the necessary framework for the rest of us to move into the biological monitoring arena and I compliment them for their leadership in this regard.

The OECD Guidance Document prepared by Chester (1995) reviews the available methods for measuring potential exposures to humans resulting from use of pesticide products. In my opinion, the sections of the Guidance Document pertaining to pharmacokinetics and biological monitoring are well written and provide an appropriate level of detail. A definition of biological monitoring is provided in conjunction with an overview of important laboratory and field considerations for study design. Reference is also made to a number of published articles for more detailed discussions of biological

*Methods of Pesticide Exposure Assessment*, Edited by
P.B. Curry *et al.*, Plenum Press, New York, 1995

monitoring. My comments are intended to support and/or supplement the discussion in the Guidance Document. I will focus on 3 aspects of biological monitoring: the importance of pharmacokinetics in biological monitoring, ethical considerations regarding biological monitoring, and generic use of biological monitoring data in quantitative exposure assessment.

## IMPORTANCE OF PHARMACOKINETICS IN BIOLOGICAL MONITORING

The potential for large interspecies differences to occur in the absorption, distribution, biotransformation and excretion of xenobiotics has been well documented (Woollen, 1993; Eberhart, *et al.*, 1991; Eberhart, *et al.*, 1989; Miyamoto, *et al.*, 1988). Furthermore, route-dependent and dose-dependent differences in the metabolism and pharmacokinetics of xenobiotics are frequently observed within the same species (Woollen, 1993; Miyamoto, *et al.*, 1988). The OECD Guidance Document makes appropriate reference to the importance of these factors and explains that their potential influence must be thoroughly evaluated before biological monitoring can be considered as a quantitative exposure assessment technique.

The following definition of biological monitoring was proposed by Woollen (Woollen, 1993) at last year's workshop in the Hague and is referenced in the OECD Guidance Document:

> Measurement of a pesticide or its metabolites in the body fluids of exposed persons and conversion to an equivalent absorbed dose of the pesticide based on a knowledge of its human metabolism and pharmacokinetics.

It is evident from this definition that a prerequisite for biological monitoring is the availability of data on a pesticide's metabolism and pharmacokinetics from studies <u>in humans</u>. The requirement for human data reflects the uncertainty associated with extrapolating metabolism and pharmacokinetic data across species. However, the OECD Guidance Document also suggests that consideration may be given to using animal metabolism and pharmacokinetic data to support biological monitoring when, for some technical or ethical reason, a human volunteer study is regarded as impracticable. This approach provides desired flexibility for individual investigators but it also raises the question of whether biological monitoring, in this context, is quantitatively superior to other monitoring techniques. Three general possibilities exist anytime an attempt is made to extrapolate metabolism and pharmacokinetic data across species:

- A pesticide's metabolism and pharmacokinetics across one or more species may be qualitatively and quantitatively different.
- A pesticide's metabolism and pharmacokinetics across one or more species may be qualitatively similar but quantitatively different.
- A pesticide's metabolism and pharmacokinetics across one or more species may be qualitatively and quantitatively similar.

From a biological monitoring standpoint, the question becomes which of these 3 possibilities is correct for any given compound. Unfortunately, the only way to determine the correct answer with the required degree of certainty is to conduct controlled clinical studies in human volunteers. The absence of human metabolism and pharmacokinetics data requires that the quantitative uncertainty associated with biological monitoring be weighed against similar uncertainty associated with the various ambient exposure monitoring techniques. As pointed out in the OECD Guidance Document, the argument may be made in specific cases that the qualitative and quantitative similarity in metabolism and excretion kinetics across several animal species supports a reasonable assumption that a similar response is expected in humans. However, it can no longer be argued in this case that the principle advantage of biological monitoring over ambient exposure monitoring is the measurement of actual, rather than potential, absorbed dose. This argument can only be accepted with an appropriate degree of certainty when biological monitoring is supported by knowledge of a pesticide's human metabolism and pharmacokinetics.

## ETHICAL CONSIDERATIONS REGARDING BIOLOGICAL MONITORING

If we accept the principle that quantitative biological monitoring requires the availability of human metabolism and pharmacokinetic data, then the issue of conducting controlled clinical studies in human volunteers must be addressed. The concept of human pesticide studies is an emotionally sensitive issue for many people in society and, in many countries, this perspective has produced a general reluctance in the scientific community to carry out these studies (Woollen, 1993). Yet, we are obligated as health and safety scientists to perform pesticide exposure/risk evaluations in the best possible manner to protect society. This dilemma opens us to criticism from both ends of the spectrum. We are criticized on the one hand for conducting human experiments with pesticides while on the other for not having relevant exposure and toxicology data to support the safe use of pesticides. In Hayes' (Hayes, 1985) review of the ethical considerations involving studies of pesticides and other xenobiotics in man, he points out that species difference in metabolism and pharmacokinetics is the justification for all studies in man. He also argues that we, as health and safety scientists, are *ethically required* to conduct human volunteer studies to support the safe use of pesticides and other non-therapeutic xenobiotics. This should be our message to society, regardless of whether we practice in industry, academia or a regulatory agency.

I am not certain whether human studies should be conducted as a matter of routine to support every available pesticide product. I am certain however, that our rationale for conducting human volunteer studies is both scientifically and ethically sound. From a scientific standpoint, controlled studies in humans are conducted to facilitate more accurate estimates of exposure which, in turn, enable more informed judgements to be made about the risks to society resulting from use of pesticide products. Without metabolism and pharmacokinetic data from humans, we must continue to make judgements based on exposure data generated using ambient monitoring techniques which have not and cannot be validated. We are obligated to develop enough data from human studies to allow us to systematically validate our ambient monitoring techniques. From an ethical standpoint, human studies using pesticides are conducted according to rigid protocols designed to protect the safety of volunteer subjects. Study protocols must be approved by independent human subjects committees after evaluating the potential risks based on data from animal studies, and volunteer subjects must give their informed consent prior to participation (Woollen, 1993; Miyamoto *et al.*, 1988; Hayes, 1985). In addition, all aspects of the studies are conducted under close medical supervision. These are the same ethical considerations which govern the conduct of human studies involving therapeutic compounds. Thus, we must convince society that the potential risks *versus* the potential benefits of human studies with pesticides are analogous to those with therapeutic agents.

The time has come for us to make a commitment to promote the development of biological monitoring as a quantitative exposure evaluation technique. It is not sufficient any longer to simply suggest that these studies offer an advantage over currently available techniques in terms of accuracy. The reality is that people are exposed, both occupationally and non-occupationally, during the use of pesticides and it is our responsibility to obtain the most appropriate data for evaluating potential risks. Thus, we must be prepared to argue that human volunteer studies with pesticides are safe and humane and that they are required to protect the interests of society. I propose that this workshop consider the future development of a position document to define the need and justification for human metabolism and pharmacokinetic data on pesticides. A document of this nature should clearly state that human studies on pesticides are recommended by an international committee of scientists from industry, academia and the regulatory agencies.

## GENERIC USE OF BIOLOGICAL MONITORING DATA

I think everyone is familiar with the concept of generic exposure estimates as they pertain to ambient exposure monitoring data i.e., the use of ambient exposure data generated for one pesticide under a given set of conditions to estimate the potential ambient exposure associated with use of a different pesticide under similar conditions (Hackathorn and Eberhart, 1985). The next session of this workshop is devoted to discussions on the development of generic databases using ambient exposure monitoring data. I believe that data from biological monitoring studies, when supported by human metabolism and pharmacokinetic data, can also be used to estimate ambient exposures for various work activities. Thus, a similar potential exists to develop a generic exposure database using biological monitoring data.

Ambient exposure monitoring is designed to measure the amount of pesticide coming into contact with a person's skin or the amount available for absorption via inhalation. Biological monitoring is designed to measure the amount of pesticide and its metabolite(s) excreted in body fluids or urine. A simple illustration of how the data from both techniques can be used to derive the same information is presented in Figure 1 and discussed below.

Data are collected in ambient exposure monitoring studies to determine the potential inhalation and dermal exposure associated with a specific work activity. These data are normalized by the mass of product handled or the duration of exposure and are considered to be generic in nature. That is, they can be used to estimate the inhalation or dermal exposure for any pesticide used in a similar manner based on the mass of product handled or the duration of exposure. These generic inhalation and dermal exposure estimates can also be compared directly to compound-specific inhalation and dermal no-observable effect levels (NOEL) from animal studies to estimate margins of safety (MOS) for each route of exposure. However, comparison to NOELs from oral dosing studies require that generic inhalation and dermal exposure estimates be corrected for absorption to estimate a systemic dose. Absorption via the inhalation route is normally assumed to be 100% whereas absorption via the dermal route is usually estimated based on compound-specific data from rat studies. Although there is no practical reason to extrapolate these data further, they could be used in conjunction compound-specific information on excretion kinetics to predict the levels of pesticide and metabolite(s) in the urine. Thus, ambient exposure monitoring data can be used to estimate the empirical data collected during a biological monitoring study.

The process of extrapolation described for ambient exposure monitoring can be reversed in the case of biological monitoring to obtain estimates of systemic dose and ambient dermal exposure. Urine samples are collected in biological monitoring studies

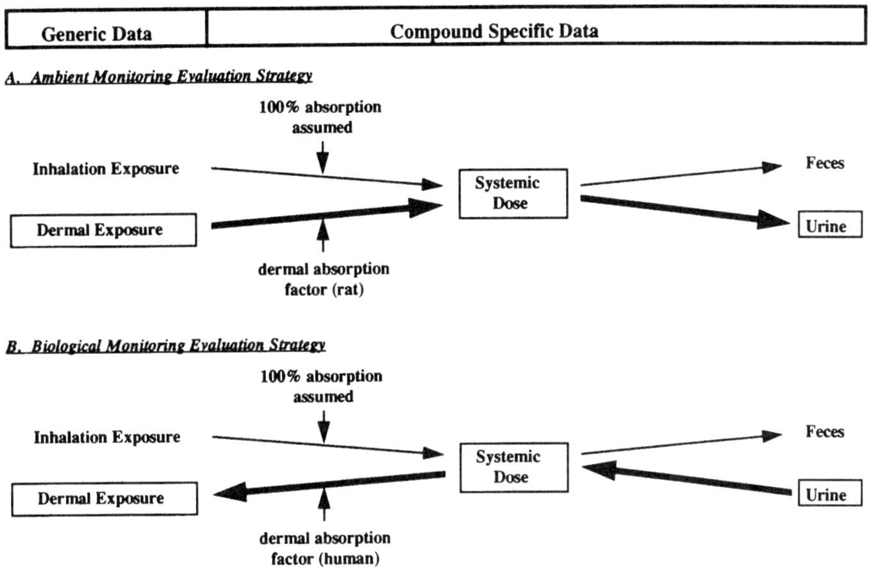


**Figure 1.** Generic versus compound-specific data for two exposure evaluation approaches. See text for discussion.

to determine the mass of pesticide and metabolite(s) excreted per day for a specific workactivity. These data are compound-specific in nature and are converted to an equivalent systemic dose of the pesticide based on knowledge of its human metabolism and pharmacokinetics. This estimate of systemic dose can be compared directly to NOELs from oral dosing studies to calculate MOS. These data can be further used in conjunction with dermal absorption data from humans to estimate ambient dermal exposures. Of course, calculation of ambient dermal exposures in this manner requires a correction to be made for the percentage of systemic dose attributable to inhalation. This can be accomplished by incorporating the measurement of ambient inhalation exposures in the field study, assuming 100% absorption, and then subtracting the estimated systemic dose via the inhalation route from the total systemic dose. At this point, the ambient dermal exposures estimated from biological monitoring data are analogous to those estimated from ambient monitoring data and can be used to prepare generic exposure evaluations.

The use of biological monitoring data to estimate ambient dermal exposures should provide more accurate estimates of *actual* dermal exposure, just as they provide more accurate estimates of *actual* systemic dose. Eventually, these data can provide a basis for quantifying the relative accuracy of the various ambient exposure monitoring techniques. An additional advantage of this approach is that these data can be incorporated into a generic database and thus, eliminate the need to conduct biological monitoring field studies for every pesticide. Even for those pesticides where it may be desirable to use dermal absorption data from human studies to reduce the uncertainty associated with animal data, the availability of generic dermal exposure data based on biological monitoring will allow accurate estimates of systemic dose to be made without conducting field studies.

## SUMMARY

The purpose of the OECD Guidance Document is to review the available methods of pesticide exposure assessment and to discuss the strengths and limitations of various evaluation strategies. The level of detail included in the sections pertaining to pharmacokinetics and biological monitoring are consistent with this purpose. However, I suggest that the following points be considered in the broader discussion of biological monitoring at this workshop:

- Biological monitoring can only be recommended as a superior quantitative exposure evaluation method when it is supported by data on the metabolism and pharmacokinetics of the pesticide in humans. In the absence of these data, the quantitative uncertainty associated with biological monitoring must be weighed against similar uncertainty associated with the various ambient exposure monitoring techniques.

- Our rationale for conducting human volunteer studies to support the development and use of biological monitoring in quantitative exposure assessment is scientifically and ethically sound. As such, consideration should be given to developing a position document defining the need and justification for human metabolism and pharmacokinetic data on pesticides.

- The potential use of biological monitoring data in generic exposure evaluations should be recognized and the feasibility of developing a generic database of ambient exposures derived from biological monitoring data should be evaluated.

## REFERENCES


Carmichael, N.G., Nolan, R.J., Perkins, J.M., Davies, R., and Warrington, S.J., 1989, Oral and dermal pharmacokinetics of triclopyr in human volunteers, *Human Toxicol.* 8:431-437.

Chester, G., 1993, Evaluation of worker exposure to, and absorption of, pesticides during occupational use and crop re-entry. *Ann. Occ. Hyg.* 37(5):509-523.

Chester, G., 1995, The Conduct of Field Studies to Evaluate the Exposure of Operators, Workers and Bystanders to Pesticides, *in:* "Proceedings of the Workshop on Methods of Pesticide Exposure Assessment, October 5-8, 1993", Ottawa.

Chester, G., Hatfield, L.D., Hart, T.B., Leppert, B.C., Swaine, H., and Tummon, O.J., 1987, Worker exposure to, and absorption of, cypermethrin during aerial application of an "ultra low volume" formulation to cotton, *Arch. Environ. Contam. Toxicol.* 16:69-78.

Chester, G., and Hart, T.B., 1986, Biological monitoring of a herbicide applied through backpack and vehicle sprayers, *Toxicol. Lett.* 33:137-149.

Dubelman, S., and Cowell, J.E., 1989, Biological monitoring technology for measurement of applicator exposure, *in:* "Biological Monitoring for Pesticide Exposure," R.G.M. Wang, C.A. Franklin, R.C. Honeycutt, and J.C. Reinert, eds. ACS Symp. Ser. No 382:240-250, American Chemical Society, Washington, D.C.

Eberhart, D., Halvorson, M., and Parkinson, A., 1989, Species differences in the *in vitro* glucuronidation of digitoxin ($dt_3$) and digitoxigenin monodigitoxoside ($dt_1$), *The Toxicologist* 9:32.

Eberhart, D., Gemzik, B., Halvorson, M., and Parkinson, A., 1991, Species differences in the toxicity and cytochrome P450 IIIA-dependent metabolism of digitoxin, *Mol. Pharm.* 40:859-867.

Hackathorn, D. R., and Eberhart, D. C., 1985, Data-base proposal for use in predicting mixer/loader-applicator exposure. *in:* "Dermal Exposure Related to Pesticide Use: Discussion of Risk Assessment," R.C. Honeycutt, G. Zweig, and N.N. Ragsdale, eds, ACS Symp. Ser. 273:341-355, American Chemical Society, Washington, D.C.

Hayes, W.J., 1985, Ethical considerations involving studies of pesticides and other xenobiotics in man, *in:* "IUPAC Pesticide Chemistry: Human Welfare and the Environment. Mode of Action, Metabolism and Toxicity," J. Miyamoto, ed., Pergamon, London, 387-394.

Miyamoto, J., Kaneko, H., Hutson, D.H., Esser, H.O., Gorbach, S., and Dorn, E., 1988, "IUPAC. Pesticide Metabolism: Extrapolation from Animals to Man," Blackwell Scientific Publications, London.

Nolan, R.J., Rick, D.L., Freshour, N.L., and Saunders, J.H., 1984, Chlorpyrifos: pharmacokinetics in human volunteers, *Toxicol. Applied Pharmacol.* 73:8-15.

Ramsey, J.D., Woollen, B.H., Auton, T.R., Batten, P.L., and Leeser, J.E., 1992, Pharmacokinetics of fluazifop-butyl in human volunteers II: Dermal dosing, *Human Exp. Toxicol.* 11:247-254.

Woollen, B.H., 1993, Biological monitoring for pesticide absorption. *Ann. Occ. Hyg.* 37(5):525-540.

Woollen, B.H., Marsh, J.R., Laird, W.J.D., and Lesser, J.E., 1992, The metabolism of cypermethrin in man: Differences in urinary metabolite profiles following oral and dermal administration, *Xenobiotica* 22 (8):983-991.

Woollen, B.H., Hart, T.B., Batten, P.L., Laird, W.J.D., Davies, D.S., and Dollery, C.T., 1991, Oral pharmacokinetics of fluazifop-butyl in human volunteers, *Human Exp. Toxicol.* 10:39-43.

# PASSIVE DOSIMETRY

# POSSIBILITIES FOR USE IN RISK ASSESSMENT

(CRITIQUE ON THE "GUIDANCE DOCUMENT" WITH RESPECT TO PASSIVE DOSIMETRY)

Wolfgang Maasfeld

Bayer AG
Plant Protection Development
Institute for Product Information and Residue Analysis
D-51368 Leverkusen

## INTRODUCTION

A clear estimation of exposure is an important step in the risk assessment for pesticides. In the "Guidance Document" prepared by Chester (1995) the available methods for measuring pesticide exposure to operators and others are reviewed and guidance is given for the determination of exposure and absorption. The "Guidance Document" provides flexibility on the approaches that can be used when conducting an exposure study.

This presentation deals with passive dosimetry. A definition given by EPA is as follows:

> "Passive dosimetry estimates the amount of a chemical impinging on the surface of the skin or the amount of the chemical available for inhalation through the use of appropriate trapping devices" (EPA, 1987).

Merely to discuss the individual methods with respect to passive dosimetry would only be a reiteration of the literature and the arguments which are already thoroughly discussed in the document. So the question arises what role passive dosimetry can play in the process of risk assessment and what has to be considered with respect to a study to serve this role.

## RISK ASSESSMENT AND PASSIVE DOSIMETRY

### The Process of Risk Assessment

In the risk assessment of pesticides with respect to operator exposure several steps have to be followed. These include on one side the hazard assessment taking into

*Methods of Pesticide Exposure Assessment*, Edited by
P.B. Curry *et al.*, Plenum Press, New York, 1995

account the NOAELs from toxicological studies and the profile of the substance. On the other side an estimation of exposure has to be performed. This can be made either using data of exposure studies performed with the product to be assessed or can be based on "generic data bases". For this estimation - which considers acute and prolonged exposure - the protective measures required by the classification and labelling of the product (cf. Council Directive 78/631/EEC) have also to be taken into account. These protective measures may already prevent hazards. Further items, among others, that have to be taken into consideration are the nature of the formulation and the specific use conditions.

### Value of Passive Dosimetry in Estimation of Exposure

The goal of the risk assessment is to ensure that a sufficient margin of safety between the estimated exposure and the NOAEL values derived from relevant toxicological studies is achieved.

It is well established that the main routes of exposure to pesticides are via dermal contact and by inhalation. As a consequence it is advisable to compare the measured or predicted dermal exposure with the results of a suitable dermal toxicological study and the same holds true for inhalation. Thus, problems arising due to route to route extrapolation (differences in absorption, biotransformation etc.) can be circumvented. This in turn requires that the exposure measurement distinguishes between dermal and inhalation exposure. And this is one advantage of passive dosimetry.

A consequence of the risk assessment may be the need for minimization of actual exposure. This "risk management" is necessary if a sufficient margin of safety is not achieved.

To serve its purpose information is needed, e.g. with respect to dermal exposure, about the appropriate body regions that are most exposed and the relative contributions of different work activities. This information again can most efficiently be gained by using passive dosimetry. The result then should be a requirement of reasonable personal protective measures that are acceptable for workers. Further measures triggered by passive dosimetry may imply changing of formulations, packaging or technologies.

## STUDY DESIGN

So the question arises how passive dosimetry should be performed in a study to estimate the dermal and inhalation exposure.

### Inhalation Exposure

A personal air sampling technique as discussed in the "Guidance Document" should be the method of first choice. Good results have been obtained with commercially available sampling tubes filled with solid adsorbents and attached to battery powered personal sampling pumps.

### Dermal Exposure

The "Guidance Document" differentiates between potential dermal exposure and actual dermal exposure. As it is desirable to get information about both, the study design should be planned in a way to monitor potential and actual exposure.

Possible methods are the patch method, the whole body method and the use of fluorescent tracers. The advantages and disadvantages of these methodologies are discussed in the literature (Durham and Wolfe, 1962; EPA, 1987; Fenske, 1990; GIFAP, 1990) and are also reviewed in the document.

The use of fluorescent tracers in combination with video imaging is promising and helpful in determining the deposition pattern. However, currently the technical availability is not that widely spread.

The patch method has the shortcoming of assuming uniform dermal deposition patterns. This can be circumvented by use of the whole body technique. Nevertheless it has to be taken into account that most exposure studies in the past have employed the patch method. A lot of data and information are available and can be used provided that appropriate data evaluation is possible. Accordingly, a pragmatic approach would be to combine both methods. The result may have the advantage that existing data can further be used and that the new data thus generated permit more flexibility and detailed information.

**Body Exposure.** Workers should wear as work clothing cotton or cotton/polyester coveralls or trousers and long sleeved shirts. This corresponds to the usual work clothing, at least in temperate climates. On the outside of these garments patches should be attached to the generally used locations (i.e. chest, back, upper arms, forearms, thighs, and lower legs). In this way, information about potential dermal exposure of different body parts can be obtained.

Beneath this clothing the workers should wear cotton undergarments (long pants and long sleeved T-shirts). In a first approach, as worst case, these results could be used for the actual exposure if work clothing would be directly worn on the skin. If this type of clothing (undergarment plus work clothing) is used as typical, a penetration factor may be taken into account for the actual dermal exposure. Further, the cumulative sampling device allows an approximate calculation of permeation through clothing and, as a consequence, also of protective action, especially if the T-shirt is sectioned, e.g., into arms and torso.

The complementary use of both methods may be an acceptable compromise combining the advantages of each method without having the disadvantages. Moreover, the workers would be dressed in a way similar to their usual clothing which in turn would also result in a "normal behaviour" during work. In contrast the practice of "normal" working methods may be more difficult when, e.g, two coveralls are used as sampling devices.

Exposure of the head region is not specially addressed in the "Guidance Document". EPA guidelines recommend either a calculation of head exposure using the shoulder, back and chest patches or a head patch. Comparison of both approaches can result in remarkable differences (Fenske, 1990).

Accordingly, the use of front and back patches attached to a cap (with or without peak, depending on the scenario) should be considered as described in the NACA guidelines (Mull and McCarthy, 1986).

**Hand Exposure.** Measurement of hand exposure is of great importance due to the high contribution to total dermal exposure. Using passive dosimetry it is suggested that workers should wear usual protective gloves (e.g., nitrile gloves), at least when handling the concentrated product or contaminated parts of the equipment. The gloves can be washed with a suitable solvent (e.g., ethanol). The results will give information about potential dermal hand exposure. If no gloves were worn the results would correspond to actual hand exposure.

Further on the hands should be rinsed with a suitable solvent (e.g., ethanol) by a standardized procedure. These results give an impression about the protective action of gloves during work or - if no gloves were worn - about actual exposure.

**General Features.** As mentioned above passive dosimetry can give valuable information on the contribution of different work steps to exposure. Therefore, when conducting a study it should be considered in advance whether mixing/loading and application should be performed with different workers. A further possibility could be monitoring of only single work activities. This may be the case when further good quality data or data for a new technique shall be implemented into a data base as mentioned in the tier approach (Carmichael, 1995).

Also the location of the patches or further additional patches may be reconsidered if detailed information of deposition patterns is available (e.g., by studies with fluorescent tracers).

## CONCLUSION

The intention of this presentation is to show what role passive dosimetry can play. It should not be understood as an argumentation against other approaches like biological monitoring.

With each study to be performed the main emphasis has to be put on the question: why is the study undertaken and how can one get the most appropriate answers.

In those cases where detailed information on the following aspects are required passive dosimetry should be considered.

In summary, passive dosimetry provides information on

→ the routes of exposure
→ the amount of exposure during different working steps and working procedures
→ the distribution of exposure for different body parts
→ the effectiveness of protective measures
→ external exposure in a standardized format suitable for use in data-bases.

Especially the last point, i.e., contribution to generic data-bases is also important. The advantage of data-bases for the development of exposure models (as proposed by Hackathorn and Eberhart, 1985) is that the variability of possible exposure is reflected, due to a broader data basis.

As the "Guidance Document" provides flexibility on the possible approaches it is recommended to discuss the arguments given and, if acceptable, to incorporate them into the document.

## ACKNOWLEDGEMENT

I would like to thank my colleagues H. Kieczka, B. Krebs and F. Mihail for helpful discussions.

## REFERENCES

Carmichael, N.G, 1995, Pesticide exposure: Overview of the tier approach, *in:* "Proceedings of the Workshop on Methods of Pesticide Exposure Assessment", October 5-8, 1993, Ottawa.

Chester, G., 1995, The conduct of field studies to evaluate the exposure of operators, workers and bystanders to pesticides, *in:* "Proceedings of the Workshop on Methods of Pesticide Exposure Assessment", October 5-8, 1993, Ottawa.

Council Directive 78/631/EEC: Council Directive of June 26, 1978, for the Approximation of the laws of the Member States Relating to Classification, Packaging, and Labelling of Dangerous Preparations (Pesticides); OJ No. L 206 of July 29, 1978.

Durham, W.F., and Wolfe, H.R., 1962, Measurement of the exposure of workers to pesticides, *Bull. WHO* 26:75.

Fenske, R.A., 1990, Nonuniformal dermal deposition patterns during occupational exposure to pesticides, *Arch. Environ. Contam. Toxicol.* 19:332.

Groupement International des Associations Nationales de Fabricants de Produits Agrochimiques, 1990, "Monitoring Studies in the Assessment of Field Worker Exposure to Pesticides", Technical Monograph No. 14, GIFAP, Brussels.

Hackathorn, D.R., and Eberhart, D.C., 1985, Data-base proposal for use in predicting mixer-loader-applicator exposure, *in*: "Dermal Exposure Related to Pesticide Use", R.C. Honeycutt, G. Zweig and N.N. Ragsdale, eds., ACS Symp. Series 273:341-355, American Chemical Society, Washington, D.C.

Mull, R., and McCarthy, J.F., 1986, Guidelines for conducting mixer-loader-applicator studies, *Vet. Hum. Toxicol.* 28:328.

U.S. Environmental Protection Agency (1987), Pesticide Assessment Guidelines, Subdivision U, Applicator Exposure Monitoring, U.S. EPA, Washington, DC.

# CRITIQUE OF THE GUIDANCE DOCUMENT AND GUIDELINES FOR THE CONDUCT OF FIELD STUDIES TO EVALUATE THE EXPOSURE OF OPERATORS, WORKERS, AND BYSTANDERS

John H. Ross

Department of Pesticide Regulation
Worker Health and Safety Branch
1020 N Street, Room 200
Sacramento, CA 95814

Concerns about chronic risks from pesticide exposure have increased in part driven by more complete toxicology databases and an increasingly wary public[1]. Risk assessments targeted at the most sensitive species at the lowest NOEL instead of mitigating acute adverse effects observable in humans under normal work conditions have fueled the need for more accurate estimates of worker exposure. A high percentage of new pesticides and an even higher percentage of "older" pesticides do not meet the acceptable risk criteria when the very conservative default exposure estimates of generic (Tier 1) studies are applied. The process of quantitative risk assessment has required scientists that monitor pesticide exposure to workers to determine delivered (absorbed) dosage. We have evolved from an industrial hygiene perspective where the work environment was monitored for ambient levels to the need to quantitate the absorbed dosage where workers themselves are monitored. The industrial hygiene measurements are still extremely valuable to evaluate environmental conditions that contribute to exposure, but these measurements frequently do not meet the demands of modern risk assessment to determine absorbed dose.

The need to mitigate worker exposure in response to calculation of excessive theoretical risk requires knowledge of both route, and ultimately absorbed dosage to determine the most effective means of exposure reduction. Traditional passive dosimetry, e.g. air pumps in the operator's breathing zone, patch or garment dermal dosimetry and handwashes provide excellent insight into route of exposure, but the number of assumptions required to translate this information into absorbed dosage frequently result in overestimates. High estimates of absorbed dosage from passive dosimetry are produced from assumptions such as everything in a handwash was available for absorption (when it may represent what was not bioavailable), extrapolation errors from patches, high percentile body surface area and low percentile body weight defaults, dermal absorption values from rats which typically overestimates humans by two to 10 fold (or 100 percent dermal absorption assumption in the absence of data), 100 percent inhalation uptake, etc.

*Methods of Pesticide Exposure Assessment*, Edited by
P.B. Curry *et al.*, Plenum Press, New York, 1995

We must make a clear distinction between exposure measurement (monitoring) and calculation (assessment). The fields of exposure monitoring and exposure assessment are both rapidly evolving. The ultimate goal of both should be to achieve the most realistic and accurate estimate of absorbed dosage for the purpose of risk assessment. Powerful new methods in exposure assessment such as the use of probability distributions in Monte Carlo simulations and estimates of target organ concentrations from physiologically based pharmacokinetics (PBPK) will become common during the next ten years. These methods will be used to provide more meaningful estimates of risk. Similarly, exposure monitoring methods are being refined with the use of human dermal absorption and human metabolism measurements to better estimate absorbed dose.

We must clearly differentiate exposure monitoring or the gathering of exposure data from exposure assessment or the estimate of absorbed dose based on the monitoring data. One is a raw data generating process and the other is data utilization and interpretation. One involves physical measurements and the other involves the mathematical and statistical use of that data. The guidance document would be strengthened if these two processes were clearly separated, because one process produces physical measurements and the other process modifies those measurements with a series of generally conservative assumptions to arrive at an estimate of absorbed dose.

The guidelines appear generally adequate in describing the need for flexibility in exposure monitoring study design dependent on the physicochemical properties of the pesticide/formulation and the manner in which it is used. However, the exposure assessment aspect is not discussed with the same thoroughness. Although the basis for body surface area is substantiated by referencing original scientific literature, the use of inhalation rates is referenced to an Environmental Protection Agency guideline which tends to use extreme upper end values of the normal range. A discussion of estimates of central tendency (geometric, arithmetic or median) and how they should be derived depending on the data distribution is lacking. The stipulation of the statistical methods to be used is a key requirement of Good Laboratory Practices. Discussion of dose amortization to reflect time to effect in a toxicologic study used to drive the risk assessment is absent. A discussion of meaningful estimates of hours worked per day, days per year, and years exposure in a lifetime are absent. While uncertainties introduced by the sampling method for clothing penetration was mentioned, there was no discussion of the mathematical method used to calculate clothing penetration. Without a common understanding of how clothing penetration is derived, it is quite possible for two individuals using the same data to arrive at different estimates of clothing penetration. Also, absent is any mention of generic exposure mitigation factors that might be applied to the results of an exposure monitoring study to test the most effective exposure reduction factors or to prospectively estimate the analytical detection limit required for a "mitigated" dosimeter.

Since the exposure assessment process can have more influence on the outcome of the risk assessment than even the design of the exposure monitoring studies, it would behoove those making absorbed dose estimates to consider both processes when designing and interpreting monitoring studies. A case in point is the choice of analytical method and limit of detection. The limit of detection must be one that yields a calculated acceptable margin of safety or risk if all the samples came out as non detects. This may seem to be a painfully simple principle, but very expensive exposure monitoring studies have been repeated because this simple guideline was not followed. For example, if the limit of detection were 10 μg per 25 $cm^2$ patch the estimated dermal dose if all patches were non detects would be approximately 8 mg.

To meaningfully use passive dosimetry data, either from a compound specific monitoring study conducted for quantitating dose in the risk assessment process, or as surrogate (Tier 1) data for a pesticide for which no compound specific monitoring data exists, specific passive dosimetry methods must be adequately validated using biological monitoring. The most direct means to do that is to conduct concurrent passive dosimetry and biological monitoring studies. This requires that the same study participants wear passive monitors (air, patch, whole body, fluorescence) during exposure with subsequent collection of (typically) urine. The guidance document offers important considerations in the design of concurrent passive dosimetry and biological monitoring studies so that the results are not compromised.

Examples of several types of concurrent passive dosimetry and biomonitoring were discussed[2,3,4,5] and their deficiencies with respect to the proposed guidelines were summarized using the attached checklist (Appendix 1). Following the guidelines will not guarantee that the results will be interpretable. Conversely not following all the guidelines does not doom the study. However, none of the studies discussed could be considered a true validation of the passive dosimetry that each employed. A true validation would constitute an agreement in absorbed dosage for both concurrent methods. Following the guidelines will improve the likelihood that a true validation can be achieved.

## APPENDIX 1

### Proposed International Guidelines: Exposure Monitoring (Checklist)

Study Design
Good Laboratory Practice (GLP) followed
Informed consent: ethical review by an HSRC
Number of subjects ≥10
Standardized dermal sampling clothing

Location and Crop
Typical equipment and/or work procedures
Sufficient area to occupy representative work day
Multiple representative worksites

Application Equipment
Full technical description

Protective Equipment
Label or regulation required PPE should be provided

Measurement of Dermal Exposure
Sampling media placement and removal aided by investigator
Integrity of sampling media checked during work day
Appropriate number and placement of dermal matrix
Handwash whenever subject wishes
Sample storage in cool boxes

Measurement of Inhalation Exposure
Samples taken in OBZ
1-2 L/min., calibrated
Cassette contains suitable analytically validated filters
Storage of media in cool boxes
Collection of only the inspirable fraction

Biological Monitoring
Appropriate metabolite for monitoring based on human metabolism study
Duration of sampling dependent on excretion kinetics
24 hr. urine collections
Subjects should shower or wash as normal
Subjects should have no further contact with test material
Two subsamples of urine taken from 24 hr. pool: 1 shipped, 1 stored

Field Storage and Stability

| | |
|---|---|
| Vehicle: | Use spray mixture from nozzle<br>Add granules or powder (pre-weighed) to sampling matrix<br>Alternatively prepare standard solutions for spiking matrix |
| Fortification Levels: | Lowest concentration = 10x LOQ<br>Fortify at multiple levels |
| Dermal Matrix: | 4 squares ~25cm each fortified at 3 concentrations each<br>4 untreated controls<br>2 squares at each concentration are stored cool, other 2 ambient |
| Handwash: | Duplicate 200 ml aliquots fortified with spray solution at 3 conc. plus control |
| Inhalation Matrices: | Duplicate filters and/or resin fortified with spray solution at 3 concentrations - connect to pumps and pull air at normal sampling rate equivalent to duration of sampling |
| Urinary Metabolites: | Spike Metabolite at 3 concentrations in duplicate 50 ml<br>Control urine spiked each day and stored under ambient worker storage conditions |
| Tank Mix: | Sample used for spiking inhalation and dermal matrices should be aliquoted in triplicate in glass vials and frozen<br>Random samples of tank mix taken throughout day |
| Weather Conditions: | Windspeed, direction, shade temperature and RH taken hourly |

## REFERENCES


1. Krieger, R.I., and Ross, J.H., Risk assessments in the pesticide regulatory process, *Ann. Occup. Hyg.* 37(5):565-578.
2. van Welie, R.T.H., van Duyn, P., Brouwer, D.H., van Hemmen, J.J., Brouwer, E.J., and Vermeulen, N.P.E., Inhalation exposure to 1,3-dichloropropene in the dutch flower-bulb culture. Part II. Biological monitoring by measurement of urinary excretion of two mercapturic acid metabolites, *Arch. Environ. Contam. Toxicol.* 20:6 (1991).
3. Weisskopf, C.P., Seiber, J.N., Maizlish, N., and Schenker, M., Personnel exposure to diazinon in a supervised pest eradication program, *Arch. Environ. Contam. Toxicol.* 17:201 (1988).
4. Fenske, R.A., Correlation of fluorescent tracer measurements of dermal exposure and urinary metabolite excretion during occupational exposure to malathion, *Am. Ind. Hyg. Assoc. J.* 49:438 (1988).
5. Formoli, R., Molinate estimated absorption based upon urinary excretion of 4-hydroxymolinate or whole body dosimetry. Review memorandum document number DPR 228-112, 133. Calif. Dept. Pest. Regul. (1993).

# Session Two

# Pesticide Exposure Databases

## SESSION TWO - PESTICIDE EXPOSURE DATABASES

## PREFACE

Session Leader: Dr. Claire Franklin

Director, Human Prescription Drugs
Health Canada
Ottawa, Ontario
Canada K1A 0L2

The goal of this session was to discuss and identify common principles between pesticide exposure databases/models that are available or being developed internationally. The concept of a database is that in lieu of exposure data from actual field studies, worker exposure for the different "use scenarios" may be estimated from information in these databases. There is tremendous potential for the use of pesticide exposure databases and the current work towards having an integrated or common database between North America and Europe is critical. The next challenge is the determination of how data from databases will be used in risk assessment. For example, what is the most appropriate estimate of the central tendency for the exposure value, the mean, the range or the 90th percentile? It is only after these parameters have been agreed upon that we will have confidence in the resultant risk estimate.

*Methods of Pesticide Exposure Assessment*, Edited by
P.B. Curry *et al.*, Plenum Press, New York, 1995

# SESSION TWO - PESTICIDE EXPOSURE DATABASES

# RAPPORTEURS' REPORT

Rapporteurs: Ron Bell[1] and France Lemieux[2]

Health Canada
[1]Chemical Evaluation Division
[2]Toxicological Evaluation Division
Ottawa, Ontario
Canada K1A 0L2

The Pesticide Handlers Exposure Database (PHED), a database developed in North America, and the European Operator Exposure Database (EUROPOEM), a predictive model being developed in Europe, were presented, compared and discussed. There was some discussion on the differences in the definitions of 'replicate' between the two databases. It was felt that resolution of the basic differences would allow for consistency between models, and the databases could then be compatible globally. There was general agreement regarding the need for consistent criteria on which to base the inclusion of exposure data in the databases. It was felt that the rejection of data should not be based on high or low exposure values but rather on the overall quality of the study. It was noted that PHED has an option whereby the user can browse through individual data points and parameters of the study and determine the acceptability of the data. Thus, the user has the option to accept or reject data.

Although differences in the European Economic Community and North America with respect to pesticide exposure criteria (e.g., acreage, crops, climate, etc.) were noted, the need to determine whether these differences affect the generic nature of the data found in both databases was identified. It was agreed that only by determining this, can harmonization of the two databases to create a global generic database proceed.

Delegates indicated that the information in the databases should be presented in a format suitable for risk-benefit analyses. It was generally agreed that in the long term, the databases could be expected to be used as a tool to make regulatory decisions.

During the discussion of the usefulness of databases, it was stated that at present, PHED could be used to determine fortification levels, the need for protective clothing and/or the level of protection required for different exposure scenarios. As well, PHED could be used as a quality assurance tool in some studies.

Two important points which were proposed by the session leader for discussion but were not addressed included algorithms and agriculture practices. These points should be addressed in the future.

*Methods of Pesticide Exposure Assessment*, Edited by
P.B. Curry *et al.*, Plenum Press, New York, 1995

# THE PESTICIDE HANDLERS EXPOSURE DATABASE (PHED): REGULATORY OVERVIEW

Alan Nielsen,[1] Patricia Curry,[2] and Tim Leighton[3]

[1]U.S. EPA, Health Effects Division
Office of Pesticide Programs
401 M Street SW
Washington, DC 20460

[2]Health Canada
Chemical Evaluation Division
Main Statistics Canada Building
Tunney's Pasture
Ottawa, Ontario, Canada K1A OL2

[3]Versar Inc.
6850 Versar Center
Springfield, Virginia 22151

## INTRODUCTION

The Pesticide Handlers Exposure Database (PHED) has been developed by the PHED Task Force in response to a NACA committee proposal that was originally presented at a 1984 American Chemical Society meeting (Hackathorn and Eberhart 1985) and further discussed in Eberhart et al., (1988). The proposal was to develop a publicly available generic database for estimating applicator exposure. The Task Force consists of representatives from Health Canada, the U.S. Environmental Protection Agency (U.S. EPA), and the National Agricultural Chemicals Association (NACA). PHED contains exposure and related data for a large number of workers engaged in mixing/loading and applying pesticide.

The database was released to the public with the approval of all Task Force members in the summer of 1992 (Federal Register 1992). PHED was released with the full acknowledgement of the limitations associated with the amount of data currently available in the system. The decision to release PHED was based on the need to rekindle support of the database, to encourage the submission of additional data, and to obtain widespread testing and scrutiny of the system.

## SYSTEM DESIGN

PHED is a predictive tool that contains measured dermal and inhalation exposure data for pesticide mixers, loaders, applicators, and flaggers. The basic assumption underlying the database is that exposure to pesticide handlers is primarily a function of the physical parameters associated with handling and applying rather than the chemical properties of individual active ingredients. The data are reported generically by type of pesticide action and formulation (i.e., not chemical specific). PHED can be used to estimate potential total exposure for a variety of scenarios including those involving different application techniques (e.g., airblast spraying) and different types of clothing worn. PHED has been developed to provide users with flexibility in designing individual exposure assessments based on their individual needs (e.g., quality assurance, replicate duration, application rate, etc.).

There are four separate data files in PHED: mixer/loader, applicator, combined mixer/loader/applicator, and flagger. The data files contain 253, 282, 224, and 42 sample replicates, respectively. PHED classifies the exposure data in each of the four PHED data files according to analytical quality assurance procedures and results. The PHED Task Force has agreed upon a grading scheme (grades A, B, C, D, or E) for inhalation, dermal, and hand exposure data points. The grades are assigned based on the results of reported quality control experiments to determine the recovery of the analyte from fortified samples. Data from three kinds of recovery experiments (i.e., laboratory, field, and storage) are used to classify exposure data.

Exposure data have not been graded based on the study design. However, data are reviewed for scientific integrity and general completeness before being accepted for entry into PHED. By basing the grading exclusively on analytical quality assurance of individual data points, the PHED Task Force has created a mechanism for capturing all valid data points, regardless of the completeness of the entire study or the quality of some of its parts. For example, a study with no hand exposure data would not generally be considered a complete study, but the data points within it for exposures to the chest, back, face, arms, and legs could still be graded and entered in PHED. By capturing all available data points, the user can define within PHED the parameters that constitute a "complete" study.

In addition to each monitoring matrix being assigned a grade, each record contains potentially 100 data points for exposure study parameters. A record represents a single worker involved in 1 day or less of a given activity. The records in PHED may include the following information: compound identification (i.e., pesticide action and formulation type); site description data; application information (e.g., application rate, cab type); personal information (e.g., years of experience); dermal and airborne exposure data; and sampling time. These parameters can be used to create user designed exposure assessments.

Statistical outputs from PHED include exposure summary reports and univariate, correlation, and regression statistics. The exposure summary reports contain the distribution type, arithmetic and geometric means, median, and coefficient of variation for each body part. Moreover, total exposure estimates are provided based on the arithmetic, geometric, and "best fit" means. The "best fit" mean is a summation of the individual body parts based on the distribution type. The "best fit" mean uses the geometric mean for lognormally distributed data, arithmetic mean for normal distribution, and the median value for "other" distributions. Univariate statistics are available for all noncoded parameters. Correlation or regression statistics can be performed on individual body part exposures or total dermal exposure. The system also allows users to create ASCII files to export data for their own use in other statistical packages.

## CURRENT USE OF PHED IN REGULATORY DECISIONS

Pesticide registration requirements of U.S. EPA require that registrants conduct studies if the pesticide of concern meets toxicity and exposure criteria that indicate potential risks to human health (U.S. EPA 1986). Health Canada requires exposure assessments for all new active ingredients, major new uses, and pesticides under official re-evaluation. Under certain circumstances regulatory agencies use surrogate data in lieu of, or in addition to, chemical specific applicator exposure field studies (Reinert et al., 1986). The U.S. EPA, Health Canada, and NACA believe that the use of an extensive, scientifically sound database is more reliable for estimating pesticide applicator exposure than the results of a single study with a limited number of replicates. By incorporating existing and future data into PHED, surrogate data may be used instead of requiring additional pesticide specific field exposure studies. This will result in substantial savings in terms of time and resources for both industry and regulatory agencies.

Historically, the U.S. EPA has relied on published literature studies as a major source of surrogate exposure data. A major limitation associated with many literature studies is the lack of adequately detailed QA/QC. Health Canada also accepts surrogate exposure data when an acceptable rationale is provided based on use patterns and application equipment, formulation type, packaging, application rate, crop, and clothing/equipment (Iyengar et al., 1993). PHED provides users with easy access to surrogate data that have been characterized based on QA/QC.

Potentially, PHED can offer several advantages to Health Canada and U.S. EPA as well as industry in estimating exposure. First, an increased number of replicates can be used in estimating exposures for some scenarios in PHED. Second, PHED eliminates some uncertainties in exposure estimates by providing consistent exposure estimates (e.g., normalization, exposure algorithms, use of actual raw data). Third, PHED offers users an easily accessible dataset for a number of exposure scenarios. Fourth, it allows regulatory agencies and industry to use the same data sets. Finally, PHED reduces cost to agencies and industry through better use of resources (e.g., identification of significant data gaps).

It is the goal of both Health Canada and U.S. EPA to consider PHED generated data in a similar manner. Consequently, these agencies have worked closely to develop the *Guidance for PHED Reporting* and the *PHED Operating Guidance*. The *Guidance for PHED Reporting* is designed to aid exposure assessors in reporting (1) appropriate subsets (e.g., application scenarios), (2) exposure data in a consistent format, (3) the details of the subset used to develop exposure estimates, and (4) significant data parameters. The *PHED Operating Guidance* outlines the major criteria that are used by the regulatory agencies to critique submissions based on PHED. The document also outlines how the agencies use PHED. The major criteria used to critique PHED generated exposure estimates include: number and duration of replicates, acceptable data grades, pesticide label requirements, normalization of exposure, extrapolation of application rates, best estimate of central tendency of exposure data, and formulation types.

PHED is currently being used in pesticide regulatory decisions by supplementing registration submittals with PHED generated exposure assessments. PHED is being used on a case-by-case basis for each registration submittal. U.S. EPA is using PHED to (1) increase the number of observations in exposure estimates and, thereby, potentially increase the reliability of the exposure assessments; (2) compare the representativeness of individual field exposure studies; and (3) verify registrant submitted PHED exposure estimates. When an appropriate subset is not available in PHED (e.g., insufficient high quality grade data for a scenario), exposure data are usually required. Specific examples of when PHED has been used by U.S. EPA include the preparation of Reregistration

Eligibility Documents (REDs), Special Reviews, and Section 18s (i.e., 1-year emergency exemptions).

## PHED LIMITATIONS FOR REGULATORY ACTIONS

Although PHED offers many advantages to regulatory agencies, industry, and researchers, the full potential of the system has not yet been realized. The three major limitations of the database are the lack of data points to adequately describe numerous exposure scenarios, insufficient high quality grade data, and the general lack of expertise among PHED users. Although a total of 801 sample replicates in the four files seem sufficient, there still are data gaps for many user created exposure scenarios. For example, an exposure study design may be created by the PHED user by extracting a subset of data for application method, cab type (four selections), replicate duration, application rate, and level/combination of type of clothing worn (e.g., gloves, coveralls, long pants/long sleeved shirts). The more restrictive the subset, the more likely an insufficient number of replicates will be available.

The second limitation, lack of high quality grade data, detracts from the ability to use PHED for regulatory decisions. Grades that are considered high quality (i.e., grade A and B for inhalation, dermal, and glove sampling techniques and grade C for hand rinse technique) are for those sampling media that meet QA/QC requirements (i.e., inclusion of acceptable laboratory/field/storage stability data). Of the 801 replicates (all media), 14 percent are grade A; 9 percent B; 51 percent C; 7 percent D; and 19 percent E. The majority of the data in PHED are graded C because even though laboratory recoveries were high (i.e., greater than 80 percent), most of the studies lacked proper field recoveries.

The third limitation for users is unfamiliarity with PHED. To use the system properly, users should have background experience in using pesticide exposure data. Users should also be aware of acceptable procedures for generating and reporting PHED exposure assessments. The previously mentioned documents, *PHED Operating Guidance* and *Guidance for PHED Reporting*, were designed to provide users with this knowledge. Both of these documents are available to all PHED users.

## PHED's FUTURE

PHED's future use as a tool for regulatory decisions hinges on the submission of additional data. Thus, the NACA Registration Committee initiated a survey to determine the number of applicator exposure studies available for submission to the database. The results of the survey indicate that there are approximately 40 to 50 exposure studies that have not been submitted for inclusion in the database. Some of the reasons that these data have not been submitted include: (1) the lack of resources for properly formatting the studies; (2) the previous inability of PHED to handle whole body dosimetry data; and (3) hesitation among submitters to sign the necessary data waiver. NOTE: All PHED submitted exposure studies are required to have a signed data compensation waiver when cited generically in PHED. U.S. EPA and NACA representatives held a meeting (June 1993) to discuss NACA participation in the database. The NACA member companies are supportive of an update in the summer of 1994 and have agreed to commit the necessary resources to submit the data.

Once updated with an additional 40 to 50 exposure studies, PHED will be a more useful tool in the regulatory decision making process. Additional data replicates will also help to further define trend analyses currently being performed (e.g., effects of personal protective equipment). Finally, the first update will allow the Task Force to better identify and prioritize data gaps and direct resources to provide a better understanding of pesticide occupational exposures. Current discussion in filling data gaps include joint industry sponsored field studies.

## CONCLUSION

PHED has been in the development stage for several years. The system is currently available and has attracted the attention of regulatory agencies, pesticide manufacturers, and researchers worldwide. What PHED potentially offers these interested parties is the ability to estimate pesticide exposures without allocating the time and resources necessary to conduct field studies.

The PHED project has illustrated international cooperation among U.S. EPA, Health Canada, and industry. The database can provide other nations with the same benefits as it does for the United States and Canada. Since exposure is assumed not to be a function of the active ingredient, but of application techniques, formulations, and other parameters, other regulatory agencies can use PHED data to evaluate pesticides.

The PHED Task Force not only encourages the submittal of North American studies, but other countries' studies as well. Greenhouse studies are especially of interest. Electronic data reporting (i.e., PHED Data Entry Diskette) is available to all data submitters. Issues that may need to be resolved before other countries' studies could be potentially incorporated into PHED are the signing of a data compensation waiver and the applicability or representativeness of application scenarios/techniques.

For further information on PHED, contact Al Nielsen/Larry Dorsey of U.S. EPA (703-305-5242), Pat Curry of Health Canada (613-957-1854), or Tim Leighton/Jeff Dawson of Versar, Inc. (703-750-3000).

## REFERENCES


Eberhart, D.C., Day, E.W., Knarr, R.D., Zimmerman, D.M., Nielsen, A.P., Reinert, J.C., and Muir, N.I., 1988, Progress in the development of a generic data base of mixer/loader-applicator exposures, *in:* "Performance of Protective Clothing: Second Symposium", ASTM STP 989, S.Z. Mansdorf, R. Sanger, and A.P. Nielsen, eds., American Society for Testing and Materials, Philadelphia, 772-775.

Federal Register, 1992, Notice of Availability of the Pesticide Handlers Exposure Database through Versar, Inc. Wednesday, June 3, 1992. Vol. 57 (107).

Hackathorn, D.R., and Eberhart, D.C., 1985, Data-base Proposal for Use in Predicting Mixer-loader Applicator Exposure, *in*: "Dermal Exposure Related to Pesticide Use", R.C. Honeycutt, G. Zweig, and N.N. Ragsdale, eds., ACS Symp. Series 273:341-355, American Chemical Society, Washington, D.C.

Iyengar, S., Curry, P.B., Nielsen, A., and Leighton, T., 1993, PHED: Where it has gone, Presented at the AgroChemical and Occupational Risk Assessment Seminar in Brussels, 1993.

Reinert, J.C., Nielsen, A.P., Lunchick, C., Hernandez, O., Mazzetta, D.M., 1986, The U.S. EPA's guidelines for applicator exposure monitoring, *Toxicol. Lett.* 33:183-191.

U.S. Environmental Protection Agency, 1986, Pesticide Asessment Guidelines, Subdivision U, applicator exposure monitoring, U.S. EPA, Washington, DC.

# A EUROPEAN OPERATOR EXPOSURE DATABASE

P. Watts[1] and W. Chen[2*]

[1]BIBRA International
Carshalton
UK

[2]DowElanco
Indianapolis
USA

## INTRODUCTION

### Regulatory Background

The authorization, placing on the market, use and control of plant protection products within the European Community is controlled by Council Directive 91/414/EEC. The importance of plant production, the role of plant protection products, the removal of national barriers to trade, the harmonization of national legislative provisions relating to the authorization of plant protection products, provisions as to data requirements and decision making criteria, and a high standard of protection for health and the environment are all provided for, or highlighted in, the Directive. Detailed rules for the evaluation of data submitted and for the authorization of preparations by individual Member States (Uniform Principles) are currently being developed.

## WORKING GROUP ON OPERATOR EXPOSURE

In connection with the development of these Uniform Principles, an ad hoc Working Group on Operator Exposure has been formed, comprised of experts from

* On behalf of the EUROPOEM Working Group: W. Chen ECPA/GIFAP (Chair); G. Chester, British Agrochemicals Association; A. J. Gilbert, Central Science Laboratory, UK; P. Y. Hamey, Pesticide Safety Directorate, UK; J. J. van Hemmen, TNO Medical Biological Laboratory, The Netherlands; S. E. Jaggers BIBRA International; K.H. Leist, Industrieverband Agrar e. V., Germany; M. R. Lynch, Pesticide Control Service, Ireland; W. Maasfeld, Industrieverband Agrar e. V., Germany; G. Milhaud, Alfort Veterinary School, France; P. Watts BIBRA International; and D. Westphal, Bundesgesundheitsamt, Germany.

*Methods of Pesticide Exposure Assessment*, Edited by
P.B. Curry *et al.*, Plenum Press, New York, 1995

France, Germany, Ireland, The Netherlands and the United Kingdom. Academia, regulatory bodies and trade associations are all represented within the Working Group (see above).

## WORKING GROUP OBJECTIVES

The major objectives of the Working Group on Operator Exposure can be summarised briefly as follows: a) to establish the scientific basis for a new and harmonised EC protocol for the prediction of operator, worker and bystander exposure to plant protection products by modelling; b) to develop a new and harmonised protocol for the conduct of field studies to evaluate the exposure of operators, workers and bystanders to plant protection products; c) to develop and construct a database containing data from European studies where exposures of operators, workers and bystanders were monitored; d) to define a tier approach in the risk assessment processes relating to the authorization of plant protection products.

## CONSTRUCTING A EUROPOEM DATABASE - A CONCERTED ACTION

This paper discusses the progress made by the Working Group relating to objective c) above, namely the development and construction of a European database of monitored operator, other worker and bystander exposures to plant protection products.

There is general agreement among scientific experts that a substantial amount of data has been generated on monitored field operator exposures to plant protection products in Europe during recent years. Much of this information at present resides in the files of individual companies, trade associations or regulatory authorities. The existing information is thus widely dispersed and not readily accessible in significant quantities either to regulatory risk assessors, industrial risk assessors or researchers. There is no single source of high quality European data on operator or bystander field exposures to plant protection products. Exposure data for various types of pesticide applications have been generated, but there is no clear awareness of the amounts of relevant exposure information for particular application types. Finally, there is no clear picture of where present and future research resources should be focused in order to plug data gaps, maximise knowledge and enhance risk assessments for operator, other worker (re-entry) or bystander exposure to plant protection products in the field.

A computer-held database of monitored operator and worker exposure studies does exist, namely the Pesticide Handlers Exposure Database (PHED). Studies comprising PHED were, in the main, generated on the North American Continent. It was considered by the Group that differences in farming and application techniques and practices might mean that the information contained in PHED may not be the most appropriate generic basis for predicting exposures in Europe.

The role that a European database could play was therefore recognised and it was agreed that the Working Group should submit to the EC Commission DG-VI (Agriculture) a Concerted Action Proposal to develop and construct a generic EUROPOEM (European Predictive Operator Exposure Model) database of monitored exposures to plant protection products within the European Community. A Proposal was drawn up and, in October 1992, submitted to DG-VI by the proposed Co-ordinator, BIBRA International, on behalf of the Group. This proposal was favourably received and in April 1993 the Co-ordinator attended a negotiation meeting at the Commission Offices in Brussels. Commission representatives invited the Group to prepare and submit a Technical Annex that succinctly summarised the Proposal and which would form a part of the eventual contract. During the production of these proceedings, the contract was signed (early 1994) and will run for 3 years from 1 January 1994.

Clearly, the value of the database would be maximised by including data from all areas of the Community. With this in mind, it is intended to adopt a flexible approach to the composition of the Group building the database, perhaps modifying this when appropriate. For example, to make the best use of Mediterranean data the Group considers it appropriate to invite experts from Mediterranean countries to participate in the relevant meetings. With this in mind, the Working Group is actively identifying appropriate expertise in the EC countries not represented on the Group at present.

## OBJECTIVES OF THE CONCERTED ACTION

The overall objective of this exercise is to develop, construct, maintain and disseminate a single, comprehensive, quality-checked and highly-accessible computerised database containing the results of EC Community-relevant monitored exposures of operators, workers and bystanders to plant protection products in the field.

### The Specific Objectives of the Project

**To Reach Agreement on Survey Forms to be Used in the Project.** These should allow data to be recorded on all of the application parameters considered to be influential in defining the exposure level of the person exposed.

**To Set Up the Database.** Initially, it is intended to use Revelation software in association with the PHED database. The market will be monitored to alert the Group to the availability of any relevant improved software. For example, an updated version of PHED is anticipated sometime during 1994. It is possible that relevant bodies in North America (the US Environmental Protection Agency (EPA), Health Canada and the US National Agricultural Chemicals Association (NACA)) will be involved in improving the available systems, and it is intended that the Group keeps abreast of any such developments. In addition, software engineers will be consulted to explore the practicalities of developing software "shells" around the Group's PHED database to allow information to be input and extracted in the units conventionally used throughout Europe, rather than the present units favoured by PHED.

**To Identify, Collate and Store Securely the Available Operator and Bystander Exposure Data.** This information is presently in the possession of diverse bodies such as agrochemical companies, agrochemical trade associations, regulatory authorities, research institutes and universities. Group participants have a strong awareness of the likely sources of relevant information, which should allow large amounts of data to be identified at the initial phase. In later phases, and for applications where no data have been found, other avenues may need to be explored for the purpose of identifying relevant data.

**To Code the Datapoints Individually.** Each datapoint represents a single monitored activity and exposure. For example, one worker carrying out a single mixing/loading exercise, with exposure being measured, is rated as one datapoint.

Coding the datapoints ensures that the relationship between the results and the originating company, the active ingredient and the formulation, is kept confidential. Only the Co-ordinator will have a record of the relation between codes and commercial information. Coding will also allow (for those using EUROPOEM data merged with PHED data) subsetting the European data for separate analysis.

**To Select Study Datapoints for Entry onto the Computerised Database.** The present basis for selection relates to the degree to which study parameters are typical of what might apply within the European Community. Priority for entry will be given to the most typical studies. Less typical studies will be given a lower priority for input.

Study design and quality will also feature in deciding whether datapoints will be selected for entry. Moreover, datapoints will not be entered if only the study summary survey forms are available, without the supporting full study being available to allow an accuracy check.

Finally, the study datapoints selected for inclusion will themselves be subject to quality grading criteria. The current thinking is that data should be graded on the basis of the reliability of the analytical data. The Group is developing selection and grading criteria.

**To Enter the Selected Datapoints onto a Suitable Computerised Database.** At present, the Group considers that the PHED database is the most appropriate to its needs. The PHED software allows datapoints to be added to one of its four existing files (applicator, mixer/loader, mixer/loader/applicator, flagger files). Data for entry onto the database will initially be taken directly from the survey forms.

**To Carry Out an Accuracy Check of the Data that have been Input.** The computerised version of each datapoint will be checked against the information contained in the original full study. Any errors in the computerised version will be corrected. Any omissions will be rectified where possible. If there are ambiguities, these will be noted and efforts made to resolve them by consulting the company/source supplying the data. Where acceptable, the computerised record will be edited to take account of any clarification the source can supply.

**To Evaluate the Usefulness of the Database in a Variety of Areas.** The data will be analysed in various ways to examine the consistency and distribution of the results, to assess the predictivity of the generic data for specific combinations of particular application parameters, to identify 'typical' parameters for possible use as surrogate values in exposure predictions using the EUROPOEM model, and to highlight datagaps. The statistical packages in the software will be sufficient for some of these analyses.

**To Identify, Agree and Rank the Study Parameters that are Critical in Determining the Level of Operator or Bystander Exposure.** It is likely that multi-regression analysis (a facility that the software package does not contain at present) will be needed to carry out this step.

**To Maintain the Database in a Live Form.** New datapoints that may become available in the future can be added to the database, enhancing its value in predicting operator exposures, in assessing potential health risks, and in focusing future research efforts.

**To Develop Methods for Dissemination of the Project Results throughout the European Community.** A critical measure of the project's success will be the degree to which interested parties can access and use the database. The Group will consider the various means by which the product can be disseminated throughout the Community and elsewhere.

## THE EUROPOEM DATABASE - CONTENT

The database will be constructed as a single, comprehensive, computerised file containing quality-selected, quality-graded, accuracy-checked data on monitored field exposures of operators, workers and bystanders to plant protection products.

In its initial form the database is expected to contain approximately 600 individual datapoints, covering exposures to boomspray applicators, air blast applicators, hand-held applicators, mixer/loaders, mixer/loader/applicators, and bystanders. In later phases, it is hoped to add further datapoints in these areas as and when they become available, and to expand the types of exposure e.g. to exposures resulting from seed treatment, greenhouse application and harvester (re-entry) exercises. Efforts will be made to identify and load datapoints relating to the use of plant protection products in all of the member states.

## THE EUROPOEM DATABASE - APPLICATIONS AND BENEFITS

The database will be a valuable addition to the total amount of scientific information available to researchers and regulatory evaluators in the European Community relating to operator field exposures to plant protection products. All of the high quality data will be available in a single, comprehensive, accuracy-checked and widely accessible computerised database.

The existence of the database will allow wider dissemination of knowledge throughout the European Community and increase the amount of high quality data that is readily available to interested parties. Moreover, awareness of the existence of relevant information will be enhanced.

The database will prove valuable to regulatory evaluators and agrochemical companies by enhancing the accuracy of predictions of likely operator exposures for new pesticides, or new applications, from a knowledge of the generic parameters, improving the scientific basis for estimating potential health risks, and establishing safety margins. It is intended that the database will be used to define the amount of relevant generic data available, which will play an important role in the proposed tier approach to risk assessment.

The existence of two databases (PHED and EUROPOEM) containing application and exposure information relevant to two different continents will allow an evaluation of how different application techniques can affect the levels of exposure.

In addition the database will be valuable to researchers. It will assist them to: a) identify datagaps (which will stimulate further research); b) focus the available research resources in areas where information is most needed; c) design and conduct future operator and bystander exposure studies; d) carry out operator and bystander risk assessments; e) develop safer formulations that result in lower exposures; f) identify application methods that result in lower exposures (i.e. safer practices) and g) select and develop better application equipment and more effective protective clothing.

## DATABASE PROGRESS

### Progress on Some Specific Objectives

**Survey Forms.** The Group has agreed on a final format for four types of survey forms: quality assurance, applicator, mixer/loader, and mixer/loader/applicator. It is believed that these survey forms encompass all of the application parameters that influence the level of operator exposure.

**Setting Up the Database.** The PHED database and the appropriate Revelation software have been purchased and set up at BIBRA International. A software engineer is providing suggestions on how to overcome difficulties relating to differences in PHED/EUROPOEM measurement units.

**Data Identification and Collation.** The Group has successfully identified about 600 relevant European datapoints. As data are selected, originating companies have been contacted and asked to supply, in strict confidence, the data to the Co-ordinator. Data are stored securely at BIBRA International.

**Coding.** Prior to entry onto the computerised database, datapoints selected for entry are being given a unique code, whose relation to commercial information is known only to the Co-ordinator. Knowledge of the assigned codes will allow subsetting of the European data.

**Selection.** The Group has selected for entry a small number (between 30-40) of datapoints on boomspray application exposure. In addition, the Group will consider some 115 mixer/loader datapoints (covering various types of application) and about 100 datapoints for boomspray mixer/loader/applicators, in order to select and prioritise for entry onto the database in the near future.

**Data Entry.** The timetable for a committed program of inputting data onto the database is highly dependent on the schedule set by the (anticipated) EC Commission contract. Since the contract was not expected to start until 1 September 1993, there has not been an opportunity to carry out a significant amount of datapoint entry. However, some 21 datapoints have now been entered, mainly to provide a preliminary assessment of the merits, suitability and potential problems of PHED. These datapoints all relate to exposure of applicators during tractor/unimog-drawn boomspray operations. The datapoints come from six different studies, carried out by three separate agrochemical companies. All six studies loaded thus far were carried out in Germany. Each study contained one to four workers carrying out one or two work cycles. Individual studies contributed between two and four datapoints. The studies were performed between 1982 and 1987. The pesticides applied were either fungicides, herbicides or insecticides and supplied as an emulsifiable concentrate, an aqueous suspension, a solution or a wettable powder. Crops included spring and summer cereals, dwarf bush beans and potatoes. Final mix concentrations varied from 0.3-11.6 g/l. The pesticides were applied to crops up to approximately 1 m in height, using booms with widths of 12-24 m. Spray volumes ranged from 100-400 l/hectare (about 10.7-42.8 US gallons/acre) and the areas treated ranged from 5-50 hectares (about 12.4-124 acres). Preliminary analyses (using the exposure calculation facilities within PHED) produced estimated total external dermal exposures (assuming no clothing, total deposition and using actual and estimated head patch data) for individual datapoints that ranged from about 52 to 31,163 μg/kg active ingredient applied (about 24 to 14,165 μg/lb active ingredient). When normalised for application time also, estimated total external dermal exposures ranged from about 27-15,715 μg/kg active ingredient/hour (see Table 1). It should be emphasized that, as yet, no attempts have been made to interpret these figures. The values generated cover a very wide range, and individual datapoints will need to be examined to establish possible reasons for the differences in estimated exposures. At this stage then, it is unclear whether outliers or differences in application parameters provide the best explanation for the range of exposure estimate values.

**Accuracy Check of Entered Data.** In each instance, the full study report has been critically assessed to confirm the accuracy and completeness of the 21 computerised

**Table 1.** Summary of estimated total dermal exposures for EUROPOEM boomspray applicators [1]

| Datapoint | µg/kg ai[2] | µg/kg ai/hr[3] |
|---|---|---|
| 9001-A-1 | 498.3 | 90.3 |
| 9001-B-1 | 272.4 | 59.4 |
| 9001-C-1 | 306.7 | 38.2 |
| 9001-D-1 | 247.0 | 77.6 |
| 9002-A-1 | 137.8 | 100.5 |
| 9002-B-1 | 52.2 | 26.7 |
| 9002-C-1 | 201.3 | 91.6 |
| 9003-A-1 | 31,162.5 | 15,715.3 |
| 9003-A-2 | 12,699.0 | 13,848.6 |
| 9004-A-1 | 5,326.8 | 1,648.2 |
| 9004-A-2 | 2,696.6 | 800.9 |
| 9004-B-1 | 211.4 | 73.7 |
| 9004-B-2 | 266.6 | 115.2 |
| 9005-A-1 | 3,736.6 | 2,114.6 |
| 9005-B-1 | 1,601.1 | 1,091.0 |
| 9005-C-1 | 28,773.9 | 7,777.0 |
| 9005-D-1 | 10,863.1 | 6,268.2 |
| 9006-A-1 | 5,825.4 | 3,602.5 |
| 9006-A-2 | 2,312.7 | 1,308.6 |
| 9006-B-1 | 3,386.1 | 4,514.3 |
| 9006-B-2 | 4,331.6 | 5,200.5 |

[1]These values were generated using the PHED estimated exposure algorithm facilities, and were calculated assuming no clothing (total deposition) and using both actual and estimated head patch data.
[2]µg/kg ai = normalised by weight of active ingredient applied.
[3]µg/kg ai/hr = normalised by weight of active ingredient applied and application time.

datapoints. The exercise has shown that data transfer from the full report to the survey forms was of a very high standard of accuracy. Liaison with the originating company has demonstrated the feasibility of clarifying ambiguities.

## SUMMARY AND CONCLUSIONS

It is widely acknowledged that the construction, maintenance and dissemination of a single, high-quality, generic computerised database of operator and bystander field exposures to plant protection products in Europe would be very useful to regulators, industrialists and researchers. It seems clear that sufficient data exist to allow the construction of such a database. With the generous assistance of the EC Commission it should be possible to construct and evaluate the database. It is important to increase awareness of the existence of the EUROPOEM database, to maintain and update the database, and to ensure that the database and the generic information contained within is as widely available as possible.

# A COMPARISON OF THE PESTICIDE HANDLERS EXPOSURE DATABASE (PHED) AND THE EUROPEAN PREDICTIVE OPERATOR EXPOSURE MODEL (EUROPOEM) DATABASE

Paul Y. Hamey*

Pesticides Safety Directorate
Mallard House, Kings Pool
3 Peasholme Green
York, Y01 2PX UK

## INTRODUCTION

Within Europe and North America there have been several independent initiatives that have established generic databases or models for predicting exposure to pesticides of workers engaged in pesticide applications. The North American Pesticides Handlers Exposure Database[1] (PHED) was the first multinational and perhaps the best sponsored attempt. Less ambitious databases or models have been assembled in the UK[2], Germany[3] and The Netherlands[4], and have been incorporated into their respective national regulatory schemes. These models have also been employed, to some extent, in other European States. The harmonisation of the regulation of plant protection pesticides within the European Community[5] requires corresponding harmonisation of the various predictive models used within Europe. Work has therefore begun using the existing PHED software to combine the individual databases, supporting the current European models, and capture further data. This venture is known as the European Predictive Operator Exposure Model (EUROPOEM) project.

Although PHED has been publicly available since 1992 the EUROPOEM initiative has not yet received official notice of the commencement of funding from the European Commission. In the absence of funding only a limited number (21) of

* On behalf of the EUROPOEM Working Group: W Chen ECPA/GIFAP (Chair); G Chester, British Agrochemicals Association; A J Gilbert, Central Science Laboratory, UK; P Y Hamey, Pesticide Safety Directorate, UK; J J van Hemmen, TNO Medical Biological Laboratory, The Netherlands; S E Jaggers BIBRA International; K H Leist, Industrieverband Agrar e. V., Germany; M R Lynch, Pesticide Control Service, Ireland; W Maasfeld, Industrieverband Agrar e. V., Germany; G. Milhaud, Alfort Veterinary School, France; P Watts BIBRA International; and D Westphal, Bundesgesundheitsant, Germany.

*Methods of Pesticide Exposure Assessment*, Edited by
P.B. Curry *et al.*, Plenum Press, New York, 1995

replicate records have been entered into the EUROPOEM database. A full comparison between the two databases is therefore not possible. However, there are a number of differences between PHED and either the approach being taken by the EUROPOEM Working Group or that adopted by existing European models. These differences are discussed below. In a recent workshop in the Netherlands, a comparision has been made between the various databases available at that time[6].

## GENERAL PRINCIPLES

There is general acceptance that a more widely representative and robust estimate of exposure can be derived from an extensive, scientifically sound and appropriate database. Conversely an estimate based on a single study with a limited number of replicates may be less representative of the levels of exposure experienced by many workers. It therefore is recognised that generic databases have a regulatory role, even when specific data are available, as a check on how representative specific exposure data are. Both PHED and EUROPOEM aim to fill this role as well as to provide estimates when specific data are not available.

PHED, EUROPOEM, and the other existing models, all have the underlying assumption that the level and distribution of potential dermal contamination to pesticides is mainly dependent on; the formulation type and handling techniques used when preparing the pesticide product for use; the type of application equipment employed; and the work practices of the individual operator. The physical and chemical properties of the active ingredient are generally not considered to be significant influences. Although in the literature examples of pesticide specific influences on potential exposure can be found[7], the wide variability in actual exposure levels is likely to mask such influences in most cases.

A possible minor difference in approach that is not apparent yet, but may be realised in future is how the databases are used. In North America the PHED database is accessed by both registrants and regulatory authorities. To ensure valid and consistent use of the database the USA Environmental Protection Agency (EPA) and Health & Welfare Canada (HWC) have defined criteria which are published in a set of guidance and standard operating procedures[8,9]. These criteria, which differ slightly between submissions for EPA and HWC, set the framework for assessments by registrants. However there is still scope for different estimates to be arrived at on the basis of valid scientific argument, so it is conceivable that different people using the PHED could arrive at different results. While the scrutiny of this would rest within the EPA or HWC, harmonisation within the European Community requires a consistent and identical approach across all EC member states. That is not to say the exposure assessment should be the same in each member state as local conditions of use may cause it to vary. It is possible, in order to realise this level of uniformity, that EUROPOEM in its final form may be more prescriptive and surrogate exposure values for different activities may be defined, as in the existing European models, rather than requiring registrants and regulators to interrogate the database for individual assessments. However, the underlying database would still be made widely available.

## SPECIFIC PRINCIPLES

### Study Design

Studies included in PHED are not graded on the basis of study design. The PHED documentation does report that data are reviewed for scientific integrity and general completeness before acceptance for entry in the database. It should be noted for a study to be regarded as complete samples do not have to be available for all body parts. EUROPOEM is following the same general criteria. The EUROPOEM Working Group wants to consider all possible exposure studies so as to avoid possible bias, but only data from well designed studies and considered to be representative of European uses will be entered into the database.

## Quality Grading

PHED grades data into classes of A to E, exclusively on analytical quality assurance criteria. These are assigned separately to inhalation, body and hand data. The minimum EPA and HWC criteria for acceptability for use in regulatory decision making are for laboratory recovery of at least 80-110% (with coefficient of variation ≤ 25 %) and with field recovery of at least 50-120%. Except for hand wash data, where the less stringent requirement is for at least 70-120% laboratory recovery (with coefficient of variation ≤ 33%) and with storage stability of 50-120%. These criteria apply no matter the age of the study, as a consequence older data without field recovery results may not be used for regulatory assessments by the EPA or HWC.

The EUROPOEM Working Group is currently discussing the approach taken within PHED and the criteria adopted by the EPA and HWC, but no conclusions have been reached. It is regarded as essential that sampling techniques and chemical analysis are adequate. However in actual practice only few studies are up to the degree of quality now required, and therefore it may not be possible to establish databases of the required size without relaxing the criteria to some extent. The Working Group is considering a preliminary pragmatic hierarchical scheme indicating criteria used to determine if the data can be included in the database. Although these discussions have only just begun the analytical data grading criteria used in PHED may be modified for EUROPOEM.

## Subsetting

To use PHED it is necessary to create a set of records representative of the conditions under consideration. For mixing and loading, the PHED guidance suggests the following as the key criteria: mixing procedure; formulation type; total amount of active ingredient handled; and packaging type. The EUROPOEM Working Group will also be investigating to see if any influence of pack size can be detected in the field as has been determined in simulated pouring tests. Another difference is that PHED does not distinguish mixing and loading for knapsack sprayers and similar equipment from mixing and loading for larger equipment such as vehicle field crop or orchard sprayers. The data in the German model show a clear difference in this aspect of handling pesticides in the field, and this difference is likely to be incorporated into EUROPOEM.

For application subsets PHED advice is that these should be based on the appropriate method of application; dose (active ingredient per area); cab type; and duration. The EUROPOEM Working Group also intends to consider if the spray volume per area has any affect in the field situation as some work has shown that the volume of contamination can depend on this parameter.

PHED guidance recommends a minimum number of 15 replicates for each body part excluding feet. Rather than being statistically derived this number is a balance between the need for a representative sample and the cost to the industry. This figure is similar to those used in existing European models. The EPA determine the minimum duration of a replicate on the basis of time required to achieve detectable residue levels. HWC judge that the duration of a replicate should represent the time that would be involved in a typical work day. The EUROPOEM Working Group also consider that replicate duration should be based on a typical work day, although it is likely that this will vary considerably across Europe. When considering different work patterns it might be appropriate to use, for example, half day replicates to estimate exposure for one scale of use, and to combine the half day replicates into single day replicates to represent a greater scale of use. However the PHED software does not allow one to combine data from an individual worker that is entered as more than one replicate over one day, into an equivalent single day's replicate.

The PHED software does allow the total amount of active substance handled, total area treated, dermal and inhalation sampling times and volume mixed or applied to be summarised. This can then be reviewed to ensure that the subset is representative of the use under consideration.

## Calculation of Exposure

A critical difference in approach between PHED and the existing European models lies in the treatment of the data in the statistical analysis of exposure. In PHED every single data point is analysed as an independent measure. This is not the approach adopted in any of the European models, and it causes the EUROPOEM Working Group some concern. An alternative approach is to calculate exposure for each individual before performing the statistical analysis. The significance of this difference is that the PHED approach gives a lower estimate of exposure than the alternative method, as is illustrated in Tables 1 and 2 respectively.

**Table 1.** Summary of PHED output for total potential dermal exposure for the initial 21 records in the EUROPOEM database

| Body part | Distribution type | Geometric mean µg/kg ai | Observations |
|---|---|---|---|
| Head (all) | Lognormal | 42.03 | 21 |
| Neck front | Lognormal | 4.30 | 21 |
| Neck back | Lognormal | 2.02 | 21 |
| Upper arms | Lognormal | 45.60 | 20 |
| Chest | Lognormal | 90.51 | 21 |
| Back | Lognormal | 77.81 | 17 |
| Forearms | Lognormal | 24.97 | 21 |
| Thighs | Lognormal | 165.52 | 21 |
| Lower legs | Lognormal | 179.02 | 20 |
| Feet | | | 0 |
| Hands | Lognormal | 271.26 | 17 |
| Total (sum of geometric means) | | 903.04 | |

## Representative Statistics

PHED uses the following statistics as point estimates of exposure; the geometric mean for lognormal, the arithmetic mean for normal, and the median for other distributions. Within Europe there have been several approaches; the UK model uses the upper limit of geometrically defined classes containing the 75th percentile; the German model uses the geometric mean; The Netherlands model uses the 90th percentile. These differences have been to some extent influenced by the different constructions of the respective models. The appropriate statistic might also be influenced by the toxicological end point and the use pattern under consideration. However ignoring such details Table 3 illustrates the significance of different statistics for the initial records in the EUROPOEM database.

**Table 2.** Individual total potential dermal exposures for the initial 21 individual records in the EUROPOEM database

| Record | µg/kg ai | Record | µg/kg ai | Record | µg/kg ai |
|---|---|---|---|---|---|
| 1 | 498.3 | 8 | 31162.5 | 15 | 1601.1 |
| 2 | 272.4 | 9 | 12699.0 | 16 | 28773.9 |
| 3 | 306.7 | 19 | 5326.8 | 17 | 10863.1 |
| 4 | 247.0 | 11 | 2696.6 | 18 | 5825.4 |
| 5 | 137/8 | 12 | 211.4 | 19 | 2312.7 |
| 6 | 52.2 | 13 | 266.6 | 20 | 3386.1 |
| 7 | 201.3 | 14 | 3736.6 | 21 | 4331.6 |
| | | | Geom. Mean 1428 | | |

**Table 3.** Representative statistics for individual total exposures from 21 records in the initial EUROPOEM database

| Statistic | Exposure µg/kg ai |
|---|---|
| 90th percentile | 12699 |
| 75th percentile | 5329 |
| Arithmetic mean | 5472 |
| Median | 2313 |
| Geometric mean | 1428 |

A limitation of the PHED software is that, although PHED has statistical analysis capability built in, it is not easily possible to get an overview of the distribution of the exposure data from which a point estimate of exposure is drawn. The EUROPOEM Working Group consider that the output from the PHED software could be improved if such facility was included, see for example Figure 1.

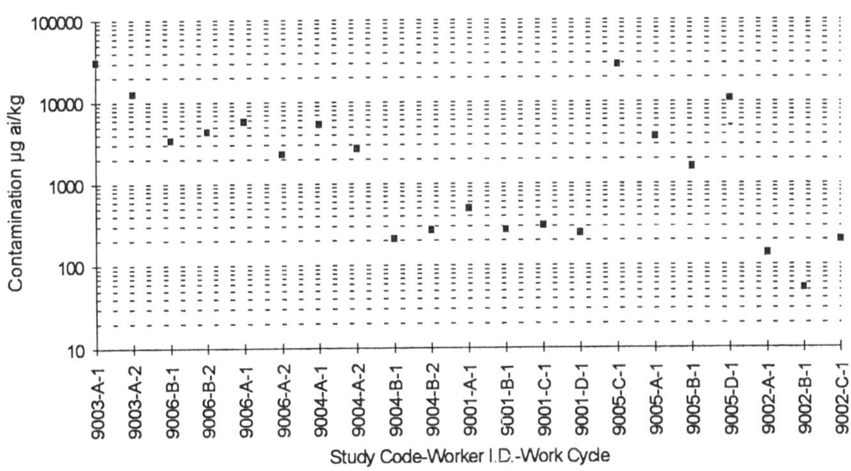


**Figure 1.** Individual total potential exposure values for the initial 21 records in the EUROPOEM database.

## Normalisation

Although PHED allows the data to be normalised on the basis of the amount of active substance handled; duration of exposure; amount of active ingredient/time; dose/area/time; the guidance for PHED reporting states that exposure should be normalised on the basis of the amount handled. Although this is the same method of normalisation as adopted in the German model the EUROPOEM Working Group have not fixed the method of normalisation. It is intended to review the available database to support any future decision. It is also recognised that where initially the range of data is limited it might be necessary to use data where the study method restricts the basis of normalisation.

**Table 4.** Summary of regression analysis of first 21 records in EUROPOEM database

| Independent variable(s) | Regression coefficient | Significance/probability |
|---|---|---|
| Single regression | | |
| Duration (hours) | 0.027 | Not significant |
| Area treated (ha) | 0.178 | Not significant |
| Amount handled (kg ai) | 0.271 | Not significant |
| Multiple regression | | |
| Amount handled (kg), area treated (ha) and duration (h) | 0.578 | 0.0018 |
| Amount handled (kg), area treated (ha), duration (h) and volume sprayed | 0.691 | 0.0005 |

As a tentative example of a possible approach that could be used in order to select the most appropriate normalisation, linear regression analysis of the first 21 data points in the EUROPOEM database was performed. Single regression with the level of total exposure as the dependent variable indicated the strongest correlation with the single independent variable of amount handled, compared to area treated and time of exposure (Table 4), although this correlation is not statistically significant. Multiple linear regression does indicate a statistically significant correlation when the amount handled, area and duration are considered together as independent variables. Furthermore including the total spray volume applied as an independent variable appears to increase the statistical significance of the analysis.

## Use of Whole Body Dosimeters

Currently, in order to analyse whole-body dosimeter data, PHED assumes uniform deposition over the entire sampling area. Therefore comparison of individual body part distribution is not possible until the PHED software is amended. The EUROPOEM Working Group has access to a significant number of studies containing whole body data so it is of interest to know how these will be analysed within PHED.

## Units

The PHED software requires data to be in American units. Limited conversion can be made when viewing the exposure calculations. For European use it is essential that all functions can be performed using standard metric values. The EUROPOEM Working Group are investigating how this might most easily be achieved. Modified summary forms have been produced to aid European workers reporting data for entry into the database.

## CONCLUSIONS

Although the EUROPOEM database has only just begun to be built as a subset of PHED there are a few significant differences that have arisen so far. Of these, the most significant is the question of should all the data points be treated as being totally independent. Related to this is the issue of which statistic should be used as a point estimate of exposure and how to indicate ranges of likely exposure. Other differences can be accommodated by the software already or of are a "cosmetic" nature.

Finally steps should be taken to improve cooperation between the two associations building the different databases so as to avoid duplication of effort.

## REFERENCES


1. PHED Reference Manual, Versar Inc, Springfield VA 22151, USA, (1991).
2. Martin, A.D. *in:* "Proceedings of Prediction of Percutaneous Penetration", R.C. Scott, R. Guy, and J. Hadgraft, ed., IBC Technical Services, London (1990).
3. Lunden, J-R., Westphal, D., Kieczka, H. *et al.* Uniform principles for safeguarding the health of applicators of plant protection products. Biologische Bundesanstalt fur Land- und Fortwirtshaft, Budesgesundheitsamt, and Industrieverband Agrar e. V. ISBN 3-489-27700-7 (1992).
4. van Hemmen, J.J., Agricultural pesticide exposure databases for risk assessment, *Rev. Environ. Contam. Toxicol.* 126:1-85 (1992).
5. Council Directive 91/414EEC, Official Journal of the European Communities, number L 327 3.12.1980.
6. van Hemmen, J.J., Predictive exposure modelling for pesticide registration, *Ann. Occup. Hyg.* 37(5): 447-586.
7. Ramaswamy, G.N., and Boyd, C.R., Fluorescent dye and pesticide penetration tested in a computerized spray chamber. Part 1. Non-woven fabrics as barriers, *Bull. Environ. Contam. Toxicol.* 51:341-348 (1993).
8. Guidance for PHED Reporting, Versar Inc, Springfield VA 22151, USA (1993).
9. Pesticide Handlers Exposure Database (PHED) Operating Guidance, Versar Inc, Springfield VA 22151, USA (1993).

# Session Three

## The Tier Approach

# SESSION THREE - THE TIER APPROACH

## PREFACE

Session Leader: Dr. Herman B.W.M. Koëter

Principal Administrator
Organisation for Economic Co-operation and Development
Environmental Health and Safety Division
2 André-Pascal
75775 Paris CEDEX 16 France

The main objective of session three was to discuss the principles of a tier approach to the use of exposure data in the regulation of pesticides. In particular, the use of surrogate data of exposure based on a generic data base was to be discussed. Further, it was considered important to discuss the amount of detail that should be included in the tier system.

In the current world economy, there is a strong drive towards harmonized standards and guidelines in many regulatory communities. In the area of pesticide regulation, we are also attempting to harmonize many approaches internationally. The harmonization of the risk assessment of pesticides is a long-standing exercise that will be ongoing for some time. An important component of this process which must be given priority is the harmonization of the use of exposure data in risk assessment. The tier approach is a first and important attempt to outline and harmonize this process.

## SESSION THREE - THE TIER APPROACH

## RAPPORTEURS' REPORT

Rapporteurs: Ron Bell and Sylvester Rozario

Health Canada
Chemical Evaluation Division
Ottawa, Ontario
Canada K1A 0L2

The structure of the session was such that first an overview of the Tier Approach was presented, followed by two critiques and a general discussion. There was general consensus regarding the concept of a tier approach for indicating the types of data required for a pesticide exposure assessment. Most agreed that a tier type system is presently being used which is dependent on toxicology, however, some individuals indicated that identifying a specific tier approach required further discussion on the criteria that would trigger each tier.

The use of the allowable occupational exposure level (AOEL) and its relevance to risk assessment was questioned. It was mentioned that the criteria for calculation of the AOEL should be defined. Whether the tier approach itself is a risk assessment process was debated. It was stated that there should be more focus on the part of the tier system that refers to the types of data requirements. It was agreed that the component of the tier system that deals with the AOEL and margin of safety would need more discussion than was possible at this workshop.

Uncertainty as to whether there are sufficient data in the generic databases to arrive at sound exposure estimates was identified. It was indicated that while there may not be sufficient data for all end use scenarios, there is an adequate amount for the more common exposure scenarios. Furthermore, there was reference to the quality of generic data required to arrive at an acceptable estimate. It was expressed that the most appropriate methods for reporting exposure values, e.g: geometric mean, $90^{th}$ percentile should be resolved.

Although the inhalation component is usually not considered to be a major element, there are instances where it does constitute a major component. Therefore, it was indicated that the tier approach should incorporate inhalation exposure.

An alternate tier system was proposed which would progress as tier 1 - potential exposure estimate; tier 2 - actual exposure estimate; and tier 3 - absorbed dose. In each of these tiers one would aim to estimate absorbed dose. There was little discussion on the specifics of each tier.

*Methods of Pesticide Exposure Assessment*, Edited by
P.B. Curry *et al.*, Plenum Press, New York, 1995

In summary, there was a general consensus on the concept of the tier approach but there were several other items that were unresolved: the AOEL and its relation to risk assessment; the incorporation of inhalation exposure into the tier approach; and the basic quality of generic databases. Much of the discussion dealt with the inclusion of the tier approach in the Guidance Document. Although there was no agreement on various aspects of the approach as introduced during this session it was agreed that the general idea of the tier approach would be outlined in the Guidance Document without mention of a specific mechanism.

# PESTICIDE EXPOSURE: OVERVIEW OF THE TIER APPROACH

Neil G. Carmichael

Rhone-Poulenc Secteur Agro
Centre de Recherche
355, rue Dostoieuski
B.P. 153
06903 Sophia-Antipolis
France

## INTRODUCTION

The tier approach which is presented here is intended as a scheme by which the hazard encountered by pesticide handlers (mixers, loader and applicators) can be assessed. Figure 1 illustrates the tiered approach under discussion. The first step in this process involves the establishment of an allowable occupational exposure level (AOEL). This value is derived in the same way as most other acceptable exposure levels, e.g., dietary (ADI) or occupational (TLV) etc. Therefore the AOEL is a number calculated from the toxicology data base by the use of an appropriate margin of safety.

The other major calculation is that of the likely exposure, as the hazard assessment scheme is based on the comparison of likely exposure with allowable exposure. Until recently this could only be performed using data from operator exposure studies in possession of the company concerned. In the last few years this situation has changed as a result of the compilation of the generic data bases which were presented in the morning session. These generic data bases offer major advantages for the commonly used application techniques as they give access to several studies and give indication of the likely variability. Once a good quality data base is established for a common application technique there would be little point in generating further exposure data of the same type.

## TIER 1

The first tier of the proposed 3 tier system is a calculation based on generic data and assumptions. Figure 2 shows the approach adopted in Tier 1.

In tier 1 the value for dermal exposure comes from a generic data base and is usually set towards the high end of the range of exposure encountered. Assumptions, mostly conservative ones, are made for extrapolation from animal to man, for the permeability of human skin, and for the effectiveness of protective measures. For example, it could be assumed that rodent and human skin were similarly permeable to

*Methods of Pesticide Exposure Assessment*, Edited by
P.B. Curry *et al.*, Plenum Press, New York, 1995

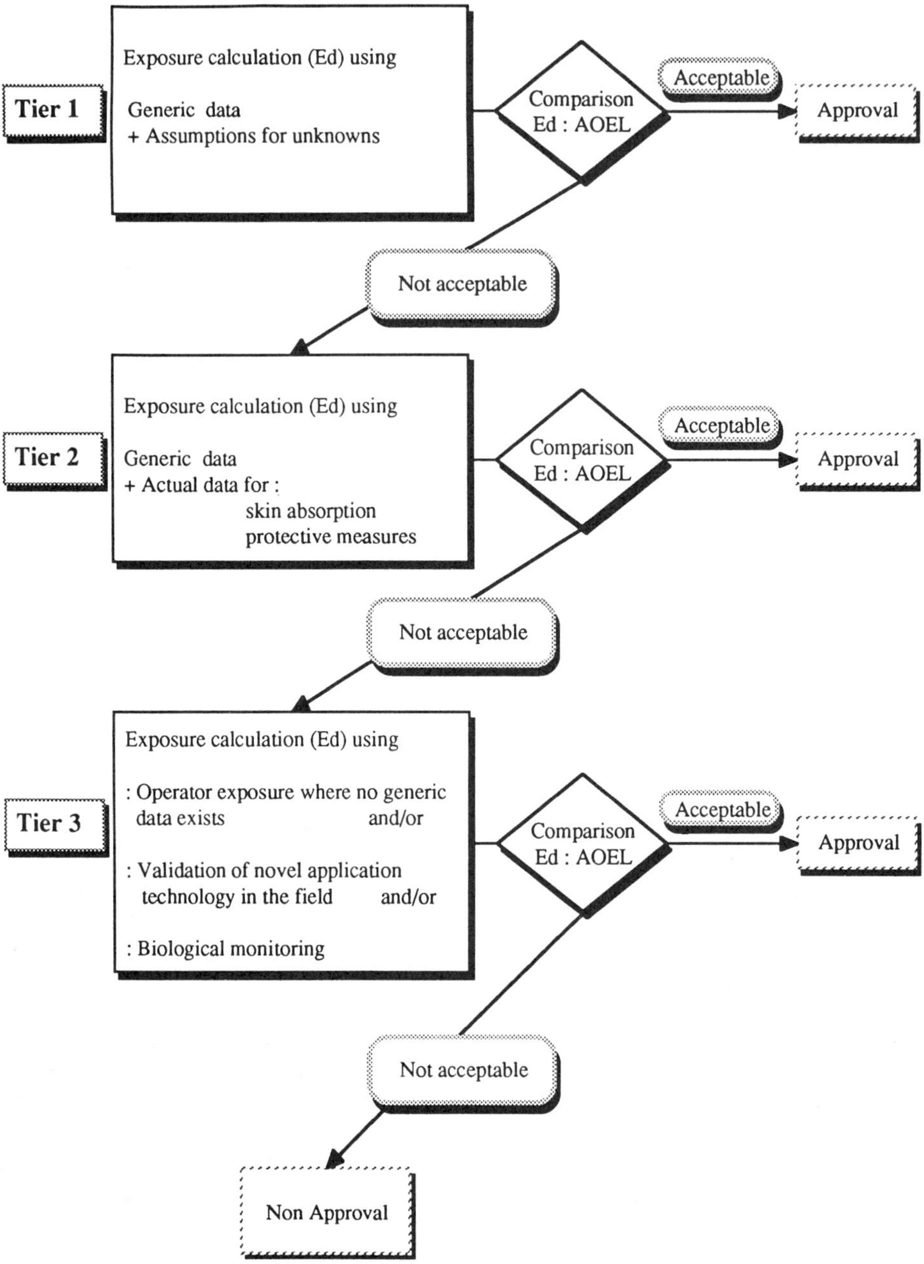


Ed = dermal exposure
AOEL = allowable occupational exposure limit

**Figure 1.** Tiered approach to applicator hazard.

the chemical in question and that gloves reduced hand contamination to 10% of the exterior contamination on the gloves. Consequently this tier 1 approach is very conservative and compounds which satisfy this assessment are likely to present minimal risk in practice.

$$\text{AOEL} = \frac{\text{NOEL}_D}{\text{MOS}}$$

$\text{NOEL}_D$ = NOEL from suitable dermal study in animals, e.g., 21 day dermal toxicity (OECD 410)
or NOEL from suitable oral toxicity study corrected for dermal absorption
if Ed < AOEL no further work is required

Ed = dermal exposure

$\text{NOEL}_D$ = dermal no effect level

MOS = Margin of safety

**Figure 2.** Tier 1.

## TIER 2

As the approach in tier 1 is very conservative there will be compounds which, on first analysis, do not achieve a sufficient margin of safety; i.e., the calculation indicates that the AOEL would be exceeded. At that point two main options become available:
1) Obtain actual data on skin penetration and/or
2) Obtain actual data on protective clothing (e.g., glove) penetration.

**Table 1.** The difference between tier 1 and tier 2

| | Tier 1 | Tier 2 |
|---|---|---|
| Exposure | generic | generic |
| Skin penetration animal | assumed | measured *in vivo* or assumed |
| Skin penetration man/animal | assumed | measured or assumed |
| Effectiveness of protective clothing | assumed | measured *in vitro* or *in vivo* or assumed |

The principle of tier 2 is to use the generic exposure data base, but to replace the assumptions used for calculating the absorbed dose with actual data. If this approach is successful there also would be no need to proceed to a further tier.

Tables 2 and 3 illustrate the type of data which might be useful in tier 2. This data was generated by the British Agrochemical Association in order to address two questions:
1) Do protective gloves work, i.e., do they give better protection than the default values which the UK model was then using?
2) Is the breakthrough time of solvents a reliable indicator of the effectiveness of gloves relative to solute (i.e., the active ingredient in the formulation)?

The results indicated that the three types of gloves tested provided very good protection against the two active ingredients studied even though two of them were penetrated fairly rapidly by xylene.

If a sufficient amount of such data were generated to be confident of its general applicability there is no reason why it could not become generic and be used in tier 1.

**Table 2**. Glove penetration study with volunteers: contamination by 0.2 ml x 12 in 6 hours

| Volunteer | Glove type | μg of active ingredient* | % of application* |
|---|---|---|---|
| Cypermethrin (10 % EC formulation) | | | |
| AS | PVC | <0.2 | <0.1 |
| AK | Nitrile | <0.2 | <0.1 |
| TP | Viton | <0.2 | <0.1 |
| AS | Nitrile | <0.2 | <0.1 |
| AK | Viton | <0.2 | <0.1 |
| TP | PVC | <0.2 | <0.1 |
| AS | Viton | <0.2 | <0.1 |
| AK | PVC | <0.2 | <0.1 |
| TP | Nitrile | <0.2 | <0.1 |
| Ioxynil Octanoate (25.5 % EC formulation) | | | |
| PS | Viton | 6.8 | 1.25 |
| GK | Viton | <0.5 | <0.1 |
| JT | Viton | <0.5 | <0.1 |
| PS | PVC | <0.5 | <0.1 |
| GK | PVC | <0.5 | <0.1 |
| JT | PVC | <0.5 | <0.1 |
| PS | Nitrile | <0.5 | <0.1 |
| GK | Nitrile | <0.5 | <0.1 |
| JT | Nitrile | <0.5 | <0.1 |

* recovered on inner cotton glove

## TIER 3

The final tier (tier 3) is reserved for situations where:
1) There is no data in the generic data base,
2) Where novel technology for application is proposed, i.e., (situation 1 above applies),
3) Where biological monitoring is able to measure the actual (i.e., compound specific) absorbed dose or biological effect of interest.

It should be re-emphasised that no purpose is served by doing a conventional worker exposure study if the generic data bases contain good quality data which can be used to predict exposure. Even if such a study showed less exposure than the existing studies it would be necessary to explain the discrepancy to justify ignoring the larger data set. However, the criterion of good quality data may be hard to verify if the data base is not open to scrutiny. In such a case it is much more useful to proceed to measuring the absorbed dose rather than external exposure.

However when new technology is introduced to reduce exposure it is to be expected that the data bases will not contain data demonstrating its effectiveness. Table 4 shows some of the technologies which have been introduced to reduce exposure.

**Table 3.** Glove penetration in vitro from EC formulations

| Permeant | Glove | Breakthrough time (minutes) | Steady-state permeation ($\mu g/cm^2/hr$) |
|---|---|---|---|
| Cypermethrin | PVC | >360 | not detected |
| | Nitrile | >360 | not detected |
| | Viton | >360 | not detected |
| Ioxynil Octanoate | PVC | >360 | not detected |
| | Nitrile | >360 | not detected |
| | Viton | >360 | not detected |
| Xylene | PVC | <45 | 15.65 |
| | Nitrile | <120 | 8.32+/-1.07 |
| | Viton | >360 | not detected |

**Table 4.** Exposure reduction technologies for agricultural chemicals

| Packaging | Formulations |
|---|---|
| Water soluble sachets | Water dispersible granules |
| Unit dose packs | Gels |
| "No-glug" jugs | Effervescent tablets |
| Metering bottles | Capsules |
| Closed system cans | Micro capsules |
| | Coated granules |

Very often a combination of packaging, formulation and application techniques can be combined to affect a major reduction of exposure compared to traditional methods. It is essential when such new technologies are introduced that there is a flexible approach to demonstrating their effectiveness. In practice this means that a study showing that the technology does decrease exposure should normally be sufficient when combined with a suitable modified calculation based on generic data bases. It should not be necessary to do a full worker exposure study under such circumstances. For example, if it can be shown that a closed system returnable can avoids all exposure during mixing and loading, it should only be necessary to calculate exposure during application.

If the safety margins obtained by calculation are still insufficient the option of biological monitoring can be considered the definitive study, but only if the conditions of applicability can be met. These conditions have already been discussed but include:
1) Known metabolic pathway,
2) Knowledge of metabolism and kinetics in man,
3) A suitable and sensitive analytical method,
4) A reliable molecule (active ingredient or metabolite) as an indicator of absorption which is available in a suitable biological matrix (preferably urine).

## CONCLUSIONS

The advantage of existing generic data bases and of their anticipated future development is that they allow the hazard assessment of agrochemicals to be simplified and avoid the generation of costly repetitive data sets. The principle is that if the assessment at a lower tier is satisfactory there is no requirement to go further. The tier system is not a list of things to do but a decision tree allowing the maximum use of already existing data and economising the use of scarce resources. Experimental data are only required where no suitable generic data exists or where conservative default values preclude a favourable evaluation.

If the proposed tier system results in large numbers of biomonitoring studies being requested it has failed in its purpose. If on the other hand it results in decisions being taken in greater confidence on the basis of larger more representative data bases then it is justifiable and to be welcomed. To this end it is imperative that the data bases are continually updated and maintained and that the quality of the data is assured.

## ACKNOWLEDGEMENT

I would like to thank the British Agrochemical Association Ltd. for permission to use the data on glove penetration and Dr. R. Scott, Dr. K. Walters and Dr. Stevenson for their contributions to this project.

# THE TIER APPROACH TO PESTICIDE EXPOSURE ASSESSMENT:

# ARE WE THERE?

Patricia B. Curry[1], Seshadri Iyengar[2], and Pamela Maloney[1]

[1]Health Canada
Chemical Evaluation Division
Ottawa, Ontario
Canada K1A 0L2

[2]Zeneca Agro
(Formerly with Health Canada)
Stoney Creek, Ontario
Canada L8G 3Z1

## INTRODUCTION

The tier approach to pesticide exposure assessment was presented and discussed at the "Workshop on Risk Assessment for Worker Exposure to Agricultural Pesticides" held in The Netherlands in May 1992. At that time there was general agreement on the merits of this approach. Theoretically, it is a logical and reasonable approach that supports the safe use of pesticides while directing attention to those areas of pesticide exposure assessment where it is most needed. This critique of the tier approach Carmichael (1995) will concentrate on the following components: generic data; assumptions on protective clothing and dermal absorption; and the allowable occupational exposure level. Figure 1 (see page 118) outlines the tier approach. The critique will address whether these components are adequately defined to allow the tier approach to be followed at this time. Lastly, personal experience in pesticide regulation will be used to identify potential problems with this approach. The purpose of this paper is to stimulate discussion of these potential problems.

## GENERIC DATA

Generic pesticide exposure databases have been created to enable the use of existing pesticide exposure data for estimating exposure to other pesticides and uses. It

*Methods of Pesticide Exposure Assessment*, Edited by
P.B. Curry *et al.*, Plenum Press, New York, 1995

is assumed that by compiling many sets of data, the resulting exposure estimate and its variability will be more representative than that obtained from a single study.

The Pesticide Handlers Exposure Database (PHED) and the European Predictive Operator Exposure Model under development are a good beginning toward the goal of generic databases. However, in using PHED, Health Canada has found that only for the most common agricultural scenarios is there sufficient good quality data at this time to estimate exposure. Thus, users should be cautioned against the assumption that the data are sufficient for all scenarios. Rather, they should be encouraged to generate data, especially for less common scenarios such as greenhouse application, indoor use, wood preservative use and turf treatment and for less common or new formulations. The databases will be useful as the basis for the tier approach as additional well designed studies with good quality data continue to be included.

Another aspect of generic exposure data that warrants discussion is the appropriate method for reporting the generic exposure value, i.e., an estimate of central tendency or the high end of the range of exposure. Dr. Carmichael pointed out that since tier 1 is a conservative approach, the exposure value should be set towards the high end of the range of exposures. However, it was apparent at the 1992 workshop in the Netherlands (Henderson *et al.,* 1992) that different countries use different estimates, ranging from the geometric mean to the 90th percentile. The general consensus on this topic at the Netherlands meeting was that the type of exposure value chosen should depend on the toxicity of the compound and the requirements of the risk assessment. For example, it was suggested that the upper limit exposure value be used for acute risk, whereas the geometric mean be used for chronic risk. In Canada, the objective is to estimate risk during typical use and consequently, an estimate of central tendency is normally used rather than the upper range. Due to the variations in study conditions, study methodologies, the personal work habits of study subjects and quality assurance and quality control, there is very large variability in the exposure estimates generated from PHED. The influence of this variability on the selection of the appropriate exposure value for risk assessment must also be considered.

## ASSUMPTIONS FOR UNKNOWNS (PROTECTIVE CLOTHING AND DERMAL ABSORPTION)

A generic database provides dermal and inhalation exposure estimates under specified conditions of use and protective measures. In order to compare an exposure estimate to an endpoint from a toxicology study conducted in laboratory animals, adjustments must be made to account for the route of administration. If the toxicology study was conducted by the dermal route, the toxicity and doses from the animal study are normally compared directly with the estimate of human dermal deposition as reported in the databases. Much work has been done in the area of dermal absorption and since it is generally accepted that rodent skin is more permeable than human skin, the direct comparison of dermal doses is reasonable. However, if the toxicology study was not conducted dermally, an assumption of dermal absorption in humans must be made in order to compare the laboratory animal toxicity to the human dermal exposure estimated from the database. Chen (1992), in a discussion of the tier approach, suggested that 10% skin penetration in humans be used as a default value. However, studies have shown that dermal absorption may be higher than 10% depending on parameters such as product formulation, concentration and conditions of use. Since this default value would be used in the conservative first tier of the approach, an assumption of 100% dermal absorption would be more reasonable when specific absorption data are unavailable.

The tier approach states that when generic data are not available for the required set of protective measures, an assumption for the effectiveness of the protective measures should be made. Research is currently ongoing to determine the protective value of clothing, particularly gloves. In extensive glove permeation work funded by the United States Environmental Protection Agency (Schwope *et al.*, 1992), results indicated that the permeation of active ingredients through various glove materials generally followed that of the carrier solution. This is in agreement with data presented from the British Agrochemicals Association (Carmichael 1995). This type of permeation data would be useful in the development of a generic data set based on carrier solvents which could be used to predict the permeation of active ingredients through various glove materials.

It was emphasized at the Netherlands workshop that additional data were needed on other types of protective clothing and measures and it was recommended that data on protective measures in actual practice be included in the pesticide registration process (Henderson *et al.*, 1992). Most glove permeation studies are conducted in controlled laboratory settings and it is unknown how these data reflect the protective value of gloves during use by pesticide handlers under field conditions. The California Environmental Protection Agency conducted a survey of the effectiveness of different protective clothing regimens and engineering controls under actual conditions of use in California and found estimates of 7-47% penetration through work clothing and 0-20% through coveralls (Thongsinthusak *et al.*, 1990). With the ongoing research in California, it may be possible to make accurate predictions on the effectiveness of protective measures in the future. It is essential that this type of research be conducted. By incorporating biological monitoring, post-registration monitoring of protective measures and health surveillance in the tier approach, this research can be used to validate assumptions made in the first tier.

## ALLOWABLE OCCUPATIONAL EXPOSURE LEVEL

The allowable occupational exposure level (AOEL) as outlined by Carmichael (1995) is based on a no-observed-effect-level (NOEL) from a suitable toxicity study and a selected margin of safety. The use of a NOEL is acceptable for threshold effects but does not consider non-threshold effects such as some types of cancer. In Canada, a weight of evidence approach incorporating quantitative risk assessment for non-threshold effects is normally used. It would be more difficult to estimate an AOEL in these circumstances. In keeping with the goal of the workshop, it is assumed that an intent of the tier approach is to allow a harmonized approach to exposure assessment. With respect to the AOEL component, it would also be necessary to harmonize and define margins of safety necessary for toxicological endpoints and use scenarios. This task is being addressed by the International Program on Chemical Safety (IPCS) in an attempt to develop a harmonized approach to health risk assessment. In Canada, it has been difficult to standardize margins of safety since many influential factors are involved in the selection of an appropriate margin of safety. These factors include the toxicological profile, the quality of the exposure data; the availability of dermal absorption data; and the contribution of risk mitigation factors such as protective clothing/equipment requirements, packaging and worker education and certification.

## OTHER COMMENTS

Inhalation exposure is not addressed in the proposed tier approach. This is likely due to the fact that in most agricultural scenarios, inhalation is often very small in comparison to dermal exposure. However, inhalation can represent a significant part of exposure in other pesticide use scenarios, e.g., fumigation and greenhouse applications. Furthermore, since it is normally assumed that 100% of inhalation exposure is absorbed, exposure by this route can comprise a significant component of the total absorbed dose. Hence, inhalation exposure should be addressed for relevant scenarios.

In Carmichael (1995), the use of skin absorption data is restricted to *in vivo* studies. Research and method development on human *in vitro* dermal absorption is ongoing (e.g., Scott *et al.*, 1992, Moody *et al.*, 1994) and the utility of this type of data should also be considered. Although Canada has not yet used this type of data in regulatory decisions, the Organisation for Economic Co-operation and Development has identified *in vitro* dermal absorption studies as a high priority for Test Guidelines.

## CONCLUSION

The tier approach to exposure assessment is a worthwhile and necessary strategy. However, it is premature to assume that there are data of adequate quality and quantity in generic databases and sufficient support for protective clothing and dermal absorption default values to allow the use of the lower tiers in the tier approach for all or even most assessments. The use of biological monitoring studies and further post-registration monitoring should be the ultimate goal for estimating pesticide exposure in cases where insufficient generic data exists. Furthermore, these studies should be used to validate the predictions made with generic databases and the assumptions made regarding protective clothing and dermal absorption.

Lastly, in order to reach a harmonized tier approach to exposure assessment it is necessary to have a harmonized approach to risk assessment. This is likely the subject of another workshop in its own right, but it must be recognized that the tier approach to exposure assessment is intimately linked to harmonized risk assessment. The standardization of safety factors for various toxicological endpoints and use scenarios is a difficult and complex task. Without the harmonization of risk assessment procedures and the standardization of safety factors it must be accepted that in using the tier approach, different countries and regulatory agencies may reach different risk decisions with the same data set.

## REFERENCES


Carmichael, N.G., 1995, Pesticide exposure: Overview of the tier approach, *in*: "Proceedings of the Workshop on Methods of Pesticide Exposure Assessment", October 5-8, 1993, Ottawa, Canada.

Chen, W.L., 1992, The harmonization of operator exposure risk assessment, Presented at the Brighton Crop Protection Conference-Pests and Diseases-1992.

Henderson, P.Th., Brouwer, D.H., Opdam, J.J.G., Stevenson, H., and Stouten, J.Th.J., 1993, Risk assessment for worker exposure to agricultural pesticides: Review of a workshop, *Ann. Occup. Hyg.* 37(5):499-507.

Moody, R.P., Nadeau, B., Chu, I., 1994, *In vivo* and *in vitro* dermal absorption of benzo[*a*]pyrene in rat, guinea pig, human and tissue-cultured skin, *J. Dermatol. Sci.* (in press).

Nielsen, A., Curry, P., and Leighton, T., 1995, The Pesticide Handlers Exposure Database (PHED): Regulatory review, *in:* "Proceedings of the Workshop on Methods of Pesticide Exposure Assessment", October 5-8, 1993, Ottawa, Canada.

Schwope, A.D., Goydan, R., Ehntholt, R., Frank, U., and Nielsen, A., 1992, Permeation resistance of glove materials to agricultural pesticides, *Am. Ind. Hyg. Assoc. J.* 53:352-361.

Scott, R.C., Batten, P.L., Clowes, H.M., Jones, B.K., and Ramsey, J.D., 1992, Further validation of an *in vitro* method to reduce the need for *in vivo* studies for measuring the absorption of chemicals through rat skin, *Fund. Appl. Toxicol.* 19:484-492.

Thongsinthusak, T., Brodber, R.K., Ross, J.H., Gibbons, D., and Krieger, R.I., 1990, Reduction of pesticide exposure by using protective clothing and enclosed cabs, Presented at the 199th American Chemical Society National Meeting, Boston, MA, April 22-27, 1990.

# QUANTITATIVE ASSESSMENT OF HUMAN PESTICIDE EXPOSURE: SOME DEFAULTS AND ASSUMPTIONS

Robert I. Krieger

University of California - Riverside
Department of Entomology
Riverside, California
U.S.A.

## INTRODUCTION

Pesticide exposure assessment is a key, dynamic element in contemporary risk assessment. The elements of the risk assessment process include hazard identification and development of dose-response relationships relevant to human health, an experimental enterprise dominated by toxicity testing in animals and the uncertainties of species-to-species extrapolations, exposure assessment in humans directed toward indirect determination of absorbed dose, and relative risk assessment for acute (margin of safety or margin of exposure) or chronic risk (excess cases of illness attributable to exposure). In either case, a health-based standard, such as the no observed adverse effect level (NOEL), provides the biological reference point for human exposure assessments.

In the Tier scheme, Carmichael demonstrates the relationship between exposure data developed with varying standards of proof. Tier 1 data derive default assumptions and generic data bases. At the other extreme, Tier 3 data represent the most complete estimate of exposure potential based upon experimental measurements and biological monitoring (Table 1).

## DEFAULTS

In order to develop transparent guidance for pesticide exposure assessment, it is centrally important to be explicit about the application of default assumptions. This should be the hallmark of Tier 1 data. Estimates that are developed to express dose (potential, estimated or absorbed) must each be based on a set of assumptions that should be fully enumerated in the guidance document. For example in Tier 1, potential dermal dose being deposited on workers, daily dermal dose reaching the skin, and absorbed daily dose are equivalent and assumed to be identical. Experimental refinement of these data

*Methods of Pesticide Exposure Assessment*, Edited by
P.B. Curry *et al.*, Plenum Press, New York, 1995

**Table 1.** Characteristics of Tier 1 and 2 Data

| Characteristic Features | Tier 1 | Tier 2 |
|---|---|---|
| Exposure[1] | potential | estimated |
| Skin penetration animal/human assumed | assumed 100% | measured in *vivo* or assumed (to 35%) |
| Effectiveness of protective clothing | assumed 90% | measured in *vitro* or in *vivo* or assumed |

[1]Expressed as absorbed dosage (μg/kg).

to reduce the number of assumptions may include assessment of clothing penetration and measurement of dermal absorption in an animal model. The result is a Tier 2 estimate of absorbed dosage which is lower and more representative of expected worker exposure than the level determined in Tier 1 (potential absorbed dosage). If investigators choose to rely upon biological monitoring to estimate dermal absorption, assumptions concerning deposition, availability of the dose (sloughing, vaporization, deposition), site-specific rates of absorption, test vehicle and pesticide formulation, and other physiological and experimental factors leave substantial scientific uncertainty.

The law of parsimony dictates that exposure estimates based upon the fewest assumptions will be the most reliable. On this basis, is it clear that Tier 3 estimates (absorbed dosage) are preferred. When exposure issues warrant, biological monitoring provides the most unambiguous exposure data. It is important to note that the exposure estimate is estimated based upon the existing foundation of metabolic and kinetic data -- and a series of assumptions based upon dose, rate and route of exposure, intraspecies and interspecies variability, and other factors unknown to investigators. Ultimately dosage is calculated as "chemical equivalents" based upon a the amount of a biomarker analyzed in a particular biological sample.

Quantitative expression of absorbed dose is the goal of exposure assessment and it is an important attribute of the tier system (Krieger *et al.*, 1992). The tier system results in development of data with varying levels of certainty with respect to human exposure. An important attribute of the system is that it can result in a clear appreciation of the working assumptions at each level and guide future research, development, and product stewardship.

## GROUPING EXPOSURE DATA

The basic scheme implies sequential development of exposure data. This scheme may be misleading, because more commonly, exposure data are developed at a particular level (tier) though a series of refinements involving varying degrees of testing, evaluation, and mitigation to achieve acceptable exposure. Movement from one level to another involves major resource decisions as well as additional scientific uncertainties. It may be more appropriate to consider the information (quantitative and descriptive) as "Level 1," "Level 2," and "Level 3" data to avoid the implication that the tiers represent a scheme for the sequential development of data.

## HANDLERS, AGRICULTURAL WORKERS AND BYSTANDERS

Pesticide use and human exposures are inextricably linked, and whether intentional, accidental, or unavoidable, at some level they can be measured and expressed as a unit of dosage (amount/body weight). On one hand, this represents a triumph of analytical chemistry because exposures are usually measured in dosages of less than µg/kg, but on the other hand, this reality alarms some people regardless of dose (Krieger *et al.*, 1992).

The same strategies of exposure assessment that are outlined for pesticide handlers (Table 1) may be applied to measurements of agricultural worker or bystander exposure. In the latter case, the investigator must be prepared to report exposure at the limit of detectability rather than "zero" if no pesticides or their associated analytes are found. Given the uncertainties associated with measuring handler and agricultural worker exposures, development of data for other groups (bystanders) who are accidentally or unavoidably exposed should proceed cautiously.

It is a relatively straightforward process to develop exposure data for agricultural workers or other persons who must contact treated crops (Krieger *et al.*, 1990). A tiered approach for development of exposure data is presented in Table 2. Dislodgeable foliar residues, work tasks, and time are the critical factors that are used to estimate the potential dermal exposure of agricultural workers. Because there are fewer mitigation options available (reentry intervals, gloves, cultural practices), it is more difficult in some cases to protect these workers from excessive exposures than it is to protect mixer/loader/applicators.

**Table 2.** Exposure-Based Field Reentry Intervals[a]

| Tier | **Dislodgeable Foliar Residue** (DFR, $\mu g/cm^2$)[b] | **Transfer Factor** (TF $cm^2/hr$)[c] |
|---|---|---|
| 1 | Limited scope, key crops | Generic[d] |
| 2 | Representative crops and use areas new technology | Passive dosimetry, skin rinse |
| 3 | Additional crops and use areas new technology | Biological monitoring |

[a] Allows development of reentry intervals for acute and chronic hazards. Since DFR is an environmental measurement, it can be assessed without harvester exposure.

[b] Environmental index will be measured when workers have contact with treated foliage.

[c] Transfer factors will be based upon exposure estimated by DFR, passive dosimetry, and biological monitoring. Absolute value will decrease Tier 1 to 2 to 3.

[d] Exposure = DFR x TF (work task dependent).

## REVIEW

The usefulness of risk assessments as a tool for the development, evaluation, and regulation of pesticide use will be determined by the dynamic balance between the protection of health and the use of chemical technologies in agriculture which are responsible for production of food and fiber. The risk assessment process requires the best possible type of use data and critically prepared exposure assessments. The process is substantially strengthened when exposures of workers are monitored to determine whether they are consistent with assessments. Such monitoring also provides insight into areas of uncertainty, which should be the subject of additional research.

Worker exposures should be monitored when a product moves into public use, and, whenever possible, the results of that work published in easily accessible journals to assure scientific evaluation and study. The follow-up monitoring may result from legislation, such as Proposition 65 in California, or from an established product stewardship program. The monitoring may take many forms, from user interviews to biological monitoring or health surveys. The overall goal is to determine the relationship between the realities of use and the assumptions of the risk assessment process.

## SUMMARY

Health-based, human pesticide exposure data are developed under several conditions which are each associated with default assumptions and scientific uncertainty. Groups of exposure data are commonly intermingled to compensate for the incompleteness of our knowledge. The three levels comprising the tier system are best considered as discrete sets of data rather than elements of a sequence or cascade of events to avoid misunderstanding and unrealistic expectations by the public and regulatory community. Data at any level (potential, estimated or absorbed dosage) may be fully adequate to support risk assessment.

Safe pesticide use requires knowledge of potential health effects, an appreciation of dose response relationships, and knowledge of the extent of human exposure, which may be obtained at three convenient levels of certainty.

## REFERENCES

Blewett, C., Edmiston, S., Fong, H., Gibbons, D., Krhieger, R., Meinders, D., O'Connell, L., Ross, J., Schneider, F., Spencer, F., and Thongsinthusak, T., 1990, Gauging pesticide exposure of handlers (mixer/loaders/applicators) and harvesters in California agriculture, *Med. Lav.* 474-479.

Krieger, R.I., Ross, John, H., and Thongsinthusak, T., 1992, Assessing human exposures to pesticides, *Rev. Environ. Contam. Toxicol.* 128:1-15.

# Session Four

# Biomarkers of Exposure

## SESSION FOUR - BIOMARKERS OF EXPOSURE

## PREFACE

Session Leader: Dr. Marco Maroni

Director
International Centre for Pesticide Safety
Via Magenta 25
Busto Garolfo (MI)
Italy 20020

The goal of this session was to discuss the usefulness of biomarkers for estimating the dose of subjects occupationally exposed to pesticides. An overview of the field as well as several state-of-the-art techniques in this field were presented.

Recent opinion surveys have found out that pesticide risk perception by the population is considerably high and that the use of pesticides is ranked in the first positions among human activities considered "at risk".

On the other hand, the assessment of the human health risk from long-term exposure to pesticides has traditionally produced little "strong" information; epidemiological studies on pesticide workers have been successful in establishing clear associations between specific exposures and health effects only for a few outcomes, and great uncertainties still exist. Even more difficulties in establishing causality appear when addressing the risk of long-term effects by pesticides in the general population. It has to be noted that the principal reason of weakness of epidemiological information resides in a poor assessment (qualitative and quantitative) of exposure.

The use of biomarkers in studies of occupational exposure to pesticides is an extremely promising tool to improve our knowledge on the risk that these compounds pose to human health. In fact they offer great opportunities to supplement traditional methods of exposure evaluation. In particular, exposure biomarkers allow the validation of the assessment of exposure made by modelling indirect information, so that exposure databases can be completed and confirmed with internal-dose databases.

The availability of new laboratory equipment and advanced techniques, such as immunochemical methods, to determine biomarkers of exposure opens new areas for research on specific risks and should encourage the conduction of health surveys on large groups of subjects.

# BIOLOGIC MARKERS: MONITORING POPULATIONS EXPOSED TO PESTICIDES

Raymond E. Grissom, Jr.

Agency for Toxic Substances and Disease Registry
Emergency Response and Consultation Branch (E32)
1600 Clifton Road, N.E.
Atlanta, Georgia 30333

Pesticides are used extensively throughout the world to control or eradicate environmental pests. Their use can be of vital importance in producing a successful crop. When properly used, pesticides do not cause adverse health effects in humans. Improper use of these substances, however, can result in adverse health effects ranging from minor dermal irritation to death.

When pesticides are being used in an attempt to eradicate environmental pests, human exposure can be evaluated using absorptive patches (Durham, 1965), examining foliar residues (Spear et al., 1965 and Spear et al., 1977), and using fluorescent imaging techniques (Fenske et al., 1986a and 1986b). Absorptive patches are frequently used by agricultural workers and others that are involved in the use of pesticides. Evaluation of the absorptive patches indicates whether exposure, particularly dermal exposure, has occurred. Evaluation of foliar residues will give an indication of the likelihood of exposure if people enter the treated area. Fluorescent imaging techniques also indicate whether dermal exposure has occurred. This procedure, however, is currently not in common use.

Exposure assessments are conducted to evaluate the potential for adverse health effects to occur. Exposure assessment, however, may not adequately address risks. Exposure assessment can document dermal exposure although dermal exposure may not accurately predict internal dose. Differences in formulation, manufacturing differences, temperature, and humidity are among the factors that may affect dermal absorption. The use of absorptive patches and fluorescent imaging techniques, and evaluation of foliar residues do not account for these factors.

Another way to show that exposure has occurred is through the use of biologic markers. Biologic markers are indicators signalling events in biologic systems or samples (NAS/NRC, 1989). For example, red blood cell (RBC) or plasma cholinesterase inhibition is an indicator of possible exposure to organophosphorus (OP) or carbamate insecticides. Detecting arsenic in urine is also a biologic marker. Biologic markers may be classified as biologic markers of exposure, effect, or susceptibility.

*Methods of Pesticide Exposure Assessment*, Edited by
P.B. Curry *et al.*, Plenum Press, New York, 1995

A biologic marker of exposure can be defined as an exogenous substance or its metabolite(s) or the product of an interaction between a xenobiotic agent and some target molecule or cell that is measured in a compartment within an organism (NAS/NRC, 1989). The most definitive biologic markers of exposure are detecting the substance of interest in a biological tissue or fluid. Detecting arsenic in the urine is a biologic marker of exposure. Detecting lead in blood is also a biologic marker of exposure. Detecting substances such as metals are always biologic markers of exposure since they cannot be metabolized or transformed into other substances. Detecting substances other than elements may require further investigation as the substance may be a parent compound or a metabolite of another substance. For example, p-nitrophenol is a metabolite of parathion (HSDB, 1993). P-nitrophenol is also a parent compound that has been used as a fungicide and a bactericide (HSDB, 1993). Detecting p-nitrophenol in urine, therefore, indicates that exposure to a substance has occurred, but does not indicate what that substance is.

A biologic marker of effect is defined as a measurable biochemical, physiologic, or other alteration within an organism that, depending on magnitude, can be recognized as an established or potential health impairment or disease (NAS/NRC, 1989). Red blood cell or plasma cholinesterase inhibition is an example of a biologic marker of effect indicating possible exposure to OP or carbamate insecticides. While it is not chemical specific, i.e., it will not implicate a specific OP or carbamate insecticide, it is usually an indicator that exposure to one of these insecticides has occurred. Biologic markers of effect are usually nonspecific. For example, gastrointestinal disturbances, headache, liver or renal dysfunction, and muscular weakness can be biologic markers of effects resulting from illness, or exposure to pesticides or other chemical substances.

Some biologic markers can be biologic markers of both exposure and effect. Tissue adducts are indicators of both exposure and effect. We may or may not be able to identify the parent substance. Methyl adducts are nonspecific; whereas, a 2,3,7,8-tetracholorodibenzo-p-dioxin (TCDD) adduct is specific.

A biologic marker of susceptibility is defined as an indicator of an inherent or acquired limitation of an organism's ability to respond to the challenge of an exposure to a specific xenobiotic (NAS/NRC, 1989). An example of a genetic biologic marker of susceptibility would be a limitation in the ability to methylate substances. Arsenic is detoxified through methylation. People with a limited capacity to methylate arsenic would have inorganic arsenic in their system longer than people who have normal or better than normal methylating capacity. Emphysema is an example of an acquired biologic marker of susceptibility. People who have emphysema may have a greater susceptibility to pesticides or other substances that affect the respiratory system.

There are numerous factors that can confound the use or interpretation of biologic markers. Pesticide formulators, loaders, applicators, harvesters, and produce processors can be exposed to pesticides. People can be exposed to pesticides if they are downwind from a pesticide application; or they may be exposed from treating their homes, lawns, and gardens with pesticides; thus, the source of the exposure may be difficult to determine using biologic markers.

If the biologic half-life of the pesticide or its metabolites is brief, the substance may have been excreted before an evaluation can be completed. Evaluating urine for arsenic needs to be performed with a couple of days after exposure since arsenic is rapidly eliminated; whereas, DDT, chlordane or other chlorinated hydrocarbon pesticides can be detected in body fat for years after exposure.

Duration and route of exposure can influence interpretation of biologic markers. Brief exposures to high levels of pesticides may produce different biologic markers than exposure to a smaller amount over a longer period of time. Pesticides that are ingested pass through the liver before entering systemic circulation. Pesticides that are inhaled or penetrate through the skin can remain in the systemic circulation for an extended period of time before being sequestered from the circulation or passing through the liver to be metabolized.

There are additional factors that can confound the use or interpretation of biologic markers. As already mentioned, biologic markers of effect tend to be nonspecific, and existing diseases may alter susceptibility to pesticide exposure. Nutritional status can confound interpretation of biologic markers. Gender, age, genetic variability, occupation, and life-style can also confound the use and interpretation of biologic markers.

Before biologic markers can be used, they must be validated in terms of their ability to assess true exposure or disease (sensitivity) and their ability to assess the lack of exposure or disease (specificity) (Dawson-Saunders and Trapp, 1990). To validate the use of a biologic measurement as a biologic marker, it is necessary to understand the relationship between the marker and the event or condition of interest. Sensitivity and specificity are critical components in the process of validation.

Sensitivity is the probability that a test result will be positive when administered to persons who have been exposed or have organ dysfunction or disease (Dawson-Saunders and Trapp, 1990). This is defined as A/A+C (see Table 1). False negatives are a problem because individuals in the false negative category have the condition of interest; however, since it has not been detected, treatment cannot be initiated and cessation of exposure may not occur.

**Table 1.** 2 x 2 Table for evaluating sensitivity, specificity, and predictive value

| | Condition Present | Condition Absent | Total |
|---|---|---|---|
| Positive Test | True Positive (A) | False Positive (B) | A+B |
| Negative Test | False Negative (C) | True Negative (D) | C+D |
| Total | A+C | B+D | A+B+C+D (N) |

Specificity relates to identifying correctly those who have not been exposed or do not have the disease or condition of interest. Specificity is defined as D/B+D (see Table 1) (Dawson-Saunders and Trapp, 1990). False positives are a problem because they can cause considerable anxiety in the individuals in this category.

Choosing a particular endpoint as evidence of abnormality affects both the sensitivity and specificity of the test. If we decrease the criteria or stringency that defines the test as positive, then we include more of those individuals who were truly affected by the toxicant (increased sensitivity); however, we simultaneously increase the number of those truly unaffected or unexposed who will test positive (decreased specificity). Careful consideration, therefore, must be given to defining where abnormality begins.

Evaluating the predictive value of a test is important for predicting health outcomes. Positive predictive value (PPV) is the probability that a person with a positive screening test has been exposed or has the disease or condition of interest and is defined as A/A+B (see Table 1) (Dawson-Saunders and Trapp, 1990). Negative predictive value (NPV) is the probability that a person with a negative screening test has not been exposed or does not have the disease or condition of interest and is expressed as D/C+D in Table 1 (Dawson-Saunders and Trapp, 1990).

The predictive value of a test is a function of the prevalence of the endpoint to be measured as well as the sensitivity and specificity of the test (Dawson-Saunders and Trapp, 1990). Prevalence is the proportion of individuals with the specified endpoint among all individuals in the population being tested and is defined as A+C/N (see Table 1). Rare events or outcomes present special difficulties when evaluating the predictive value of a test. Sensitivity and specificity are independent of the prevalence of the disease or condition of interest while predictive value varies with disease or condition prevalence. Therefore, the prevalence of the exposed population among the screened population will determine the predictive value of the test (Dawson-Saunders and Trapp, 1990).

Biologic markers of effect are not discrete entities. They occur as a continuum (see Figure 1) (Schulte, 1988). Obviously, exposure has to occur before the events to the right of exposure in Figure 1 can occur. A small or brief exposure may not result in an internal dose, the dose may have been excreted or sequestered before evaluation occurred, or the internal dose may be below the detection limit of the test procedure being employed. Detection of an internal dose does not indicate that a biologically effective dose is present. A biologically effective dose is a dose that results in pesticide at the site of toxic action. The dose may be metabolized, excreted, or in some other way removed from circulation before any early biological effects can occur. As the dose is increased, the biologically effective dose will progress to early biological effects. An example of an early biologic effect is a decrease in plasma or RBC cholinesterase activity resulting from exposure to an OP or a carbamate insecticide. A slight decrease in activity indicates that an early biological effect has occurred; however, clinical symptoms may not be observed because of the abundance of the esterase. Carbon tetrachloride may cause an increase in plasma levels of hepatic enzymes although hepatic function may not be altered. As the dose of the OP or carbamate insecticide, or carbon tetrachloride is increased, altered structure or function will occur followed by disease or death.

Clinically, we may not be able to observe the progression from exposure to other end points along the continuum. For example, exposure may result in death. The internal dose, biologically effective dose, early biological effect, and altered structure or function occurred; however, the dose was of such magnitude that exposure and subsequent death were the only events clinically observable. Exposure may be followed by internal dose, biologically effective dose, early biological effect, or altered structure or function.

Exposure —> Internal Dose —> Biologically Effective Dose —> Early Biological Effect —> Altered Structure or Function —> Disease or Death

**Figure 1.** Biologic marker continuum.

The Agency for Toxic Substances and Disease Registry (ATSDR) has produced Toxicological Profiles for many pesticides. Toxicological Profiles for chlorinated hydrocarbon insecticides include aldrin/dieldrin, chlordane, DDT/DDE/DDD, endrin/endrin aldehyde, heptachlor/heptachlor epoxide, hexachlorocyclohexanes (lindane), mirex, and toxaphene. Toxicological Profiles for metals that have been used as pesticides include arsenic, copper, lead, mercury, and tin. Toxicological Profiles for chemicals used as fumigants include bromomethane, carbon disulfide, carbon tetrachloride, cyanide, and 1,2-dichloropropane. Toxicological Profiles for impurities found in pesticide include chlorodibenzo-p-dioxins and TCDD. A Toxicological Profile has been produced for methyl parathion. Toxicological Profiles for volatile organic compounds (VOCs) that have been used as solvents for pesticides include isophrone, methylene chloride, and xylenes.

Each profile contains information about biologic markers. The information in Figure 2 was taken from ATSDR's Toxicological Profile for Lead (ATSDR, 1993). Section 2.5 contains generic information about biologic markers. Sections 2.5.1 and 2.5.2 contain specific information about biologic markers of exposure and effect, respectively, resulting from environmental exposures to lead. Other profiles contain specific biologic marker of exposure and effect information about the substance discussed in the profile.

2.5 BIOMARKERS OF EXPOSURE AND EFFECT
2.5.1 Biomarkers Used to Identify or Quantify Exposure to Lead
2.5.2 Biomarkers Used to Characterize Effects Caused by Lead

**Figure 2.** Biologic marker information in toxicological profiles.

ATSDR is continuing its efforts to develop, validate, and use biologic markers. ATSDR has developed biologic marker panels for evaluating renal, hepatic, neurological, immune, and respiratory function. The Agency is in the process of validating these biologic marker panels in studies conducted by ATSDR's Division of Health Studies (DHS).

The Agency will continue to evaluate biologic markers through the Agency's exposure registry program. The purpose of the registry is to assess the long-term health effects of long-term exposure to low levels of environmental contaminants. If a substantial population has been exposed to a hazardous substance, an exposure registry will be established.

One of the goals of the registry is to establish a database that will furnish the information needed to generate appropriate and valid hypotheses for future activities such as epidemiologic studies. The registry is not a definitive study. Cause and effect relationships cannot be established using only registry-based information. However, the results of the data analysis will identify reported health outcomes that should be considered for future activities.

Data collected in the registry will assist scientists and physicians in developing, validating, and using biologic markers. The information collected for each member of the registry will include environmental and demographic data, smoking and occupational history, and self-reported responses to 25 general health status questions. The files for each chemical-specific registry are established when baseline data are collected and are maintained and regularly updated by ATSDR. Information derived from the registry will be published and made available to the public.

ATSDR's Division of Health Assessment and Consultation (DHAC) may be involved in the selection of sites where biologic marker panels will be used. The Emergency Response and Health Consultation Branch is involved in emergency response activities and responding to specific questions about potential adverse health effects at sites where hazardous materials are present. Health Consultations are brief documents that can be prepared and released rapidly. In the event that emergency response activities or Health Consultations identify a major problem, a Health Assessment may be prepared by DHAC's Health Assessment Branch. Health Assessments are detailed documents that look at a much broader scope than Health Consultations. If a significant threat to human health is found to exist, DHS may conduct an epidemiological study using the biologic marker panels developed by the Agency. Through this type of action, the Agency is employing and validating its biologic marker panels.

ATSDR's Division of Toxicology (DT) will continue to implement the substance specific research on biologic markers as described in Section 2.9 of the toxicological profiles. The Division of Toxicology is responsible for identifying data needs for substances for which it has prepared toxicological profiles. Data needs have been identified for biologic markers for these substances. As mentioned earlier, toxicological profiles have been prepared for numerous pesticides and substances associated with pesticides. Biologic markers data needs for these substances have been identified, and DT is in the process of filling these data needs.

## REFERENCES


Agency for Toxic Substances and Disease Registry (ATSDR), 1993, "Toxicological Profile for Lead", U.S. Public Health Service, Agency for Toxic Substances and Disease Registry, Atlanta, Georgia, NTIS No. TP-92-12.

Dawson-Saunders, B., and Trapp, R.G., 1990, "Basic and Clinical Biostatistics", Appleton and Lange, Norwalk, Connecticut/San Mateo, California.

Durham, W.F., 1965, Pesticide exposure in man and animals, *Arch. Environ. Health* 10:842-846.

Fenske, R.A., Leffingwell, and Spencer, W.F., 1986a, A video imaging technique for assessing dermal exposure I. Instrument design and testing, *Am. Ind. Hyg. Assoc, J.* 47:764-770.

Fenske, R.A., Leffingwell, and Spencer, W.F., 1986b, A video imaging technique for assessing dermal exposure II. Fluorescent tracer testing, *Am. Ind. Hyg. Assoc. J.* 47:771-775.

Hazardous Substances Data Bank (HSDB), 1993, U.S. Department of Health and Human Services Data Base, National Institute of Health, National Library of Medicine, Bethesda, Maryland 20894, USA.

National Academy of Sciences/National Research Council (NAS/NRC), 1989, "Biologic Markers in Reproductive Toxicology", National Academy of Sciences/National Research Council, National Academy Press, Washington, D.C.

Schulte, P.A., 1988, A conceptual framework for the validation and use of biologic markers, *Environ. Res.* 48:129-144.

Spear, R.C., Popendorf, W.J., Leffingwell, J.T., Milby, T.H., Davies, J.E., and Spencer, W.F., 1965, Field workers response to weathered residues of parathion, *J. Occup. Med.* 19:406-410.

Spear, R.C., Popendorf, W.J., Spencer, W.F., and Milby, T.H., 1977, Worker poisoning due to parathion residues, *J. Occup. Med.* 19:411-414.

# USING IMMUNOCHEMICAL METHODS TO ANALYZE FOR BIOMARKERS OF EXPOSURE

Shirley J. Gee[1], Anne D. Lucas[2] and Bruce D. Hammock[1]

[1]Departments of Entomology and Environmental Toxicology
University of California
Davis, California 95616-8584

[2]Food and Drug Administration
Center for Devices and Radiological Health
12709 Twinbrook Parkway (HFZ-112)
Rockville, MD 20852

## INTRODUCTION

Studies assessing the exposure of workers, consumers, and others to pesticides are among the most costly aspects of assuring the safety of a pesticide. The analysis of samples is a significant portion of that cost (sample collection, sample preservation, transport, sample preparation, instrumental analysis time and data reduction). Information is presented here about an analytical technique that may be useful in providing data at a reduced cost. Immunochemical techniques used in the analysis of drugs and hormones in the clinical laboratory provide analytical information for a few dollars per analysis, whereas typical analytical costs for a pesticide in an environmental matrix may run from \$50-\$1000 per sample depending on the analyte, matrix and analytical method.

**Table 1.** Disciplines involved in the development of immunochemical techniques

| | |
|---|---|
| Hapten synthesis | Antibody characterization |
| Hapten conjugation to carrier proteins | Assay development |
| Immunization | Assay validation |

Immunochemical techniques, like other analytical methods, utilize a selective detector; that detector is an antibody. The antibody is a reagent that is designed, characterized and validated. Table 1 describes the basic methodology involved in the development of these antibody-based assays. It is beyond the scope of this report to describe these procedures in detail. It is, however, important to point out that a multidisciplinary approach is needed. Synthetic organic chemistry and protein chemistry are needed for hapten synthesis and conjugation. Biochemistry and immunochemistry are important to raising and characterizing antibodies and assay development. Analytical chemistry plays a large role in the validation by integrating sample preparation methods and standard analysis methods (i.e., gas-liquid chromatography or high performance liquid chromatography) with immunochemical analysis. Further discussion can be found in several reviews (Harrison et al., 1988; Jung et al., 1989; Hall et al., 1990; Van Emon and Lopez-Avila, 1992).

## Advantages and Disadvantages

There are several advantages to immunochemical techniques:

1) Sensitivity - assays can usually detect nanogram quantities of analyte. Two examples are measuring atrazine in soil extracts or food (Schneider and Hammock, 1992; Wittmann and Hock, 1993) and metolachlor in water (Lawruk et al., 1993). Current pesticides that use very low application rates, such as sulfonylureas, are also driving the need for highly sensitive assays.

2) Selectivity - antibodies can be highly selective. Assays have been developed to detect parent compound alone, parent and metabolites (Feng et al., 1992) or a class of compounds (Wie and Hammock, 1984). Some antibodies have been designed to distinguish among chiral isomers (Wing et al., 1978).

3) Speed of analysis - the actual length of instrumental analysis time per sample can be measured in minutes and multiple samples can be processed in parallel. A large portion of analysis time is devoted to sample preparation. For immunoassay analysis, sample preparation can be very minimal. For example, a pesticide can be measured in urine by adjusting the pH of the sample and then adding it to the analysis (Lucas et al., 1993). Extraction and purification steps may be eliminated or greatly reduced which then also results in decreased solvent usage and disposal.

4) Cost effectiveness - the per sample costs can be low due to decreased sample preparation and parallel sample processing. In the clinical field, where immunoassay is a primary analytical technique, each sample may cost only a few dollars to run. The ability to handle large samples loads may allow researchers to conduct studies that require a large number of samples, for example to address the question of the degree of individual variability that will be encountered in a field exposure study. There are strong economies of scale with immunoassays. Since exposure studies usually involve many samples in a uniform matrix, immunoassays are very inexpensive.

5) Applicability - this technique has been applied to a wide variety of compound types. It is easiest to design assays for larger molecular weight, water-soluble, hydrolytically stable, non-volatile compounds (i.e., paraquat and sulfonylureas; Van Emon et al., 1986; Schlaeppi et al., 1992). However, other compounds can be accommodated. Thus assays have been reported for small molecular weight compounds such as lipophilic pyrethroids (Stanker et al., 1989), hydrolytically unstable carbamates (Marco et al., 1993), organophosphates (Skerritt et al., 1992) and volatile thiocarbamate herbicides (Gee et al., 1988). The technique is especially applicable to the analysis of polar metabolites including conjugates as diagnostic metabolites.

6) Adaptability - probably one of the most attractive advantages is the adaptability of the technology. Once reagents have been made, they can be formatted in a variety of ways such as a yes/no field test kit, highly quantitative laboratory test and anything in between. Field test kits, for example, can be used to provide timely data, and may also be the most expedient way to measure those compounds that are unstable to transport and storage. In addition, the antibodies may be applied to development of

biosensors (Wong and Ahmed, 1992) or used in the preparation of samples as in immunoaffinity chromatography (Hayashi et al., 1990; Katz and Brady, 1990).

There are, of course, also disadvantages to any technique:

1) Sensitivity - the high sensitivity possible with immunoassays may create problems in detecting very low exposure levels. Samples may need to be diluted 100 to 1000 times in order for the concentration to fall within the linear range of the standard curve. This may mean that error associated with large dilutions decrease the utility of the assay as a highly quantitative method. Such sensitivity can, however, be adjusted to reasonable levels by the developer of the assay. In regulatory situations, where a worst-case scenario is figured into risk evaluations, high sensitivity can prove beneficial.

2) Interferences - as with other analytical techniques, immunoassays are susceptible to specific interferences (termed cross-reactivity) and non-specific interferences, for example due to the matrix. These must be carefully characterized in order for the immunoassay to be useful. However, the low cost and speed of immunoassays make it simple to develop quantitative tests for cross-reactivity and matrix effects and then to take measures to correct for these effects.

3) New technology - as a new technology, time must be invested to train the analytical chemist in its use. Training manuals such as one written in collaboration with the U.S. Environmental Protection Agency may serve a useful introduction (Gee et al., 1994). Immunoassay is a relatively new and expanding technology in the field of exposure assessment to environmental chemicals. However, immunoassay has been in use for following the pharmacokinetics of pharmaceuticals for decades. Like other mature technologies, there are many manuals in the clinical area available that are directly applicable to worker exposure.

4) Reagent availability - since this is a new technology, reagents are not readily available. Only fairly recently have antibody-based test kits become available commercially.

5) Large sample load required - to justify the cost of development, there must be a large sample load for analysis.

6) Multi-analyte analysis - in general, immunoassays are single analyte methods. They are not easily applied, for example, to evaluating a hazardous waste site. However, this is not likely a problem in exposure assessment studies, since the analytes are usually known. It is relatively straightforward to use an indicator metabolite for a class of compounds such as the mercapturate for most triazine herbicides (Lucas et al., 1993), substituted nitrophenols for many organophosphate insecticides (Li et al., 1991) or m-

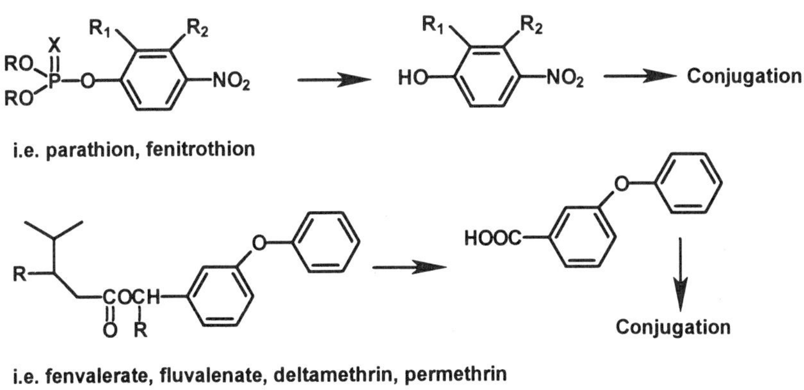


Figure 1. Examples of metabolites as indicators of exposure to parent pesticides.

phenoxybenzoic acid for most pyrethroid insecticides (Wengatz, work in progress; Figure 1). It is also possible to develop an assay for an indicator class of metabolites. For instance antibodies selective for mercapturates of lipophilic compounds could indicate exposure to a variety of electrophiles while 8-oxo-2'-deoxyguanosine immunoassays are used as urinary indicators of DNA damage in humans (Ames et al., 1993).

### History

Immunochemical methods were first described in 1945 when Landsteiner proposed that antibodies could bind selectively to small molecules (termed haptens) when they were attached to a larger carrier molecule (Landsteiner, 1945). This "hapten-specific" response was explored by Yalow and Berson in the late 1950's and resulted in an immunoassay that was used to monitor plasma insulin in humans (Yalow and Berson, 1959; Yalow and Berson, 1960). This work set the stage for the rapid advancement of immunochemical methods for clinical use.

The first pesticide antibodies were not described until 1970 when Centeno and Johnson developed antibodies that bound malathion (Centeno and Johnson, 1970). Shortly thereafter, radioimmunoassays were developed for aldrin and dieldrin (Langone and van Vunakis, 1975). Up until this time, immunoassays were generally precipitation assays or used radioisotopes as labels. In 1972, Engvall and Perlman reported the first use of enzymes as labels and coined the term "enzyme-linked" immunosorbent assay or ELISA (Engvall and Perlmann, 1972). In 1980, Hammock and Mumma described the potential for ELISA for the analysis of pesticides (Hammock and Mumma, 1980). Since that time the number of papers describing immunoassays for pesticides has grown dramatically and a journal devoted to this area is being published (Food and Agricultural Immunology, Carfax Publishing Company, Abingdon, United Kingdom).

## APPLICATION OF IMMUNOCHEMICAL METHODS TO PESTICIDE RESIDUE ANALYSIS

Any research endeavour requiring analysis for pesticides may be amenable to using immunochemical techniques. Table 2 is a listing of areas in which immunoassays may be used. Dr. van Hemmen's presentation mentioned the need for a field test kit for monitoring dislodgable foliar residues prior to reentry. Compliance monitoring and environmental fate studies are two other examples of potential use for this technology. It could be used in formulation analysis to verify quality of the formulation and to avoid potential cross contamination of products when switching production at a plant. Food and feed safety are becoming more important and likely precipitate the analysis of a larger number of samples. With the historical use of immunoassays in clinical medicine for monitoring drugs and hormones in urine and blood, it seems that use of this technology for monitoring biomarkers of exposure is most applicable. Here we want to be able to monitor parent compounds or metabolites in urine. Immunoassays are among the few techniques available for monitoring other biomarkers, such as adducts of DNA, haemoglobin and albumin and also one of the few techniques available to monitor the new generation of biological pesticides (Cheung and Hammock, 1988; Hammock, 1988) and products of recombinant DNA research (McDiarmid and Strickland, 1990). In many cases, immunoassays may be best suited to screening large sample loads for ranking samples prior to a secondary confirmation method (Lee et al., 1990). This is one example that demonstrates that immunochemical techniques should be considered among the variety of analytical methods available for solving problems in analytical chemistry.

**Table 2.** Analytical problems for which immunoassay may be useful

| | |
|---|---|
| Reentry monitoring | Residue analysis |
| Environmental monitoring | Formulation analysis |
| Food & feed quality | Biomarkers of exposure |

## PRINCIPLES OF IMMUNOCHEMICAL ANALYSIS

Immunochemical methods can be formatted in a variety of ways. Figure 2 is a schematic representation of how the components of an immunoassay can be assembled. A variety of formats are described in the literature (Voller et al., 1976; Tijssen, 1985).

The reactants are in a state of equilibrium as shown in Figure 3. Thus immunoassays are governed by the Law of Mass Action and are physical assays, rather than bioassays, even though biological reagents are utilized. On the positive side, immunoassays are highly quantitative and reproducible. The resulting data can be analyzed by a variety of mathematical techniques. However, since immunoassays are not bioassays, an immunoassay response cannot be evaluated in terms of biological effects unless the experiments supporting such extrapolation have been performed.

The absorbance readings resulting from the analysis are plotted vs the log of the concentration of the analyte. Figure 4 shows a model standard curve. These curves are described by the 4-parameter logistic equation of Rodbard (Rodbard, 1981) and unknowns can then be extrapolated from a curve such as this.

The above concepts have been applied to the development of a variety of "formats". In one test kit format, antibodies are immobilized on polystyrene test tubes and dropper bottles are used to deliver reagents. Washing steps are conducted using water from a tap. Color development can be compared to a color chart or alternatively read in a field portable spectrophotometer. A quantitative laboratory test may consist of

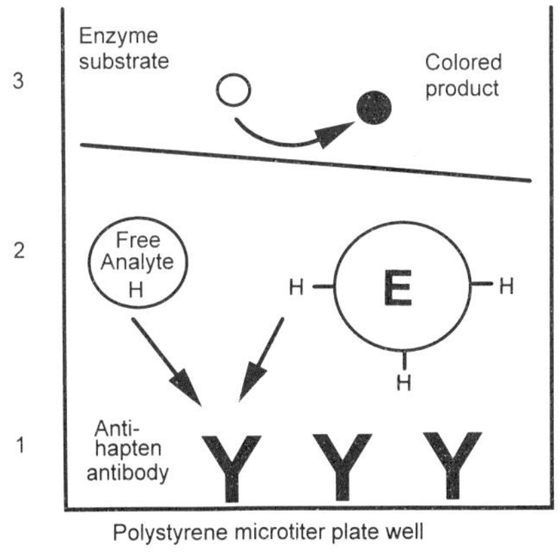


**Figure 2.** The anti-pesticide antibody is immobilized to a solid phase (in this case, the well of a 96-well microtiter plate). The sample or standard containing analyte and the "label" are added to the well. In this case, the label is an enzyme with a covalently bound analyte-mimic. The free analyte and the analyte-mimic on the enzyme compete for a fixed amount of anti-analyte antibody on the solid phase. Unbound reactants are washed out of the well. Substrate for the enzyme is then added, and color development monitored. The more analyte that is present in the sample, the less label that can bind to the antibody. Conversely, the less analyte that is present in the sample, the more label that can bind to the antibody and thus more color is developed. In this competitive format then, the color development is inversely proportional to the concentration of analyte.

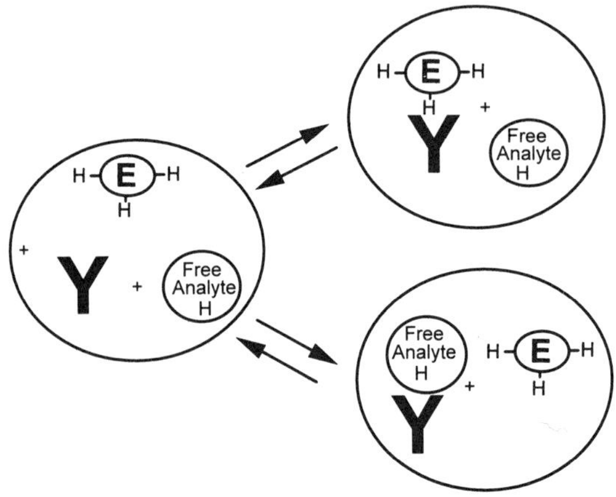


**Figure 3.** Schematic of the equilibrium reactions occurring during the immunoassay. The circle on the top right depicts the binding of the enzyme label (**H-E**) to the anti-pesticide antibody (**Y**). The circle on the bottom right depicts the binding of the analyte (**H**) to the anti-pesticide antibody. The circle on the far left depicts the free reactants in solution.

a microtiter plate reader and multichannel pipettor. With this instrumentation a single analyst may be able to process 100-200 samples per day. This degree of simplicity then may provide a powerful tool to developing countries for conducting very sophisticated exposure assessment studies. Finally, immunoassays may be formatted such that all steps are handled by a computer assisted robotic system. Such systems are currently used for mass screening for plant pathogens (Dewey et al., 1991).

## DETECTION OF ATRAZINE MERCAPTURATE AS A BIOMARKER OF EXPOSURE USING ANTIBODIES

As a step in the validation process, the immunoassay is utilized to determine the analyte concentration in a variety of matrices. "Blank" matrices may be spiked and recoveries determined. Determining the concentration of analyte in a series of samples obtained in the field and comparison of these data to those obtained by a second instrumental method is ideal. A series of triazine assays was developed in this laboratory

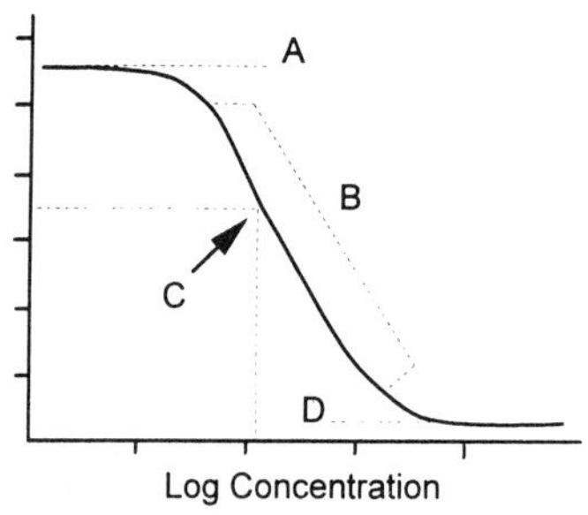


**Figure 4.** Model standard curve generated by enzyme immunoassay. The concentration of analyte is plotted versus the absorbance. The sigmoid curve is described by a 4-parameter logistic equation where A and D are the upper and lower asymptote, respectively, B is the slope and C is the midpoint of the curve.

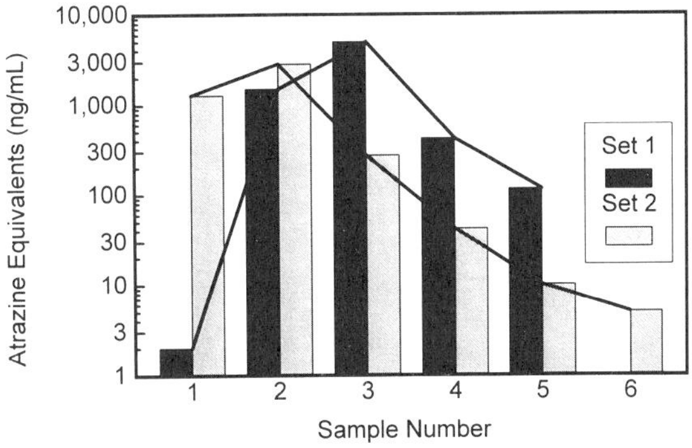


**Figure 5.** Concentration of "atrazine" found by immunoassay, in human urine samples from volunteers with a known exposure to atrazine.

for the purpose of monitoring atrazine, simazine and prometon in groundwater (Goodrow et al., 1990; Harrison et al., 1991; Karu et al., 1991; Lucas et al., 1992; Schneider and Hammock, 1992). In an effort to validate the assay method for atrazine in urine, we obtained some urine samples from volunteers who had a known exposure to atrazine from the Worker Health and Safety Branch of the California Department of Food and Agriculture. These same samples had been previously analyzed by gas liquid chromatography (GC) for atrazine.

Figure 5 shows the results of that analysis. Both sample sets showed a large concentration of "atrazine" by the immunoassay method. This immunoreactive material was present in measurable amounts for up to six days. A rough estimate of the half-life of the material was calculated to be 24 hours. The GC analysis of these same samples indicated that in no sample was atrazine present at greater than 8 ng/mL (ppb). This antibody was not cross reactive to several known breakdown products of atrazine, such as the N-dealkylated metabolites or hydroxyatrazine. An examination of the structures of the pesticide mimic used to raise antibodies (Figure 6) led us to postulate that the immunoreactive material was the N-acetyl cysteine derivative of atrazine (atrazine mercapturate). Reevaluation of the samples with an antibody which detected atrazine, but not its mercapturate yielded data that agreed with the very low levels of atrazine detected by GC.

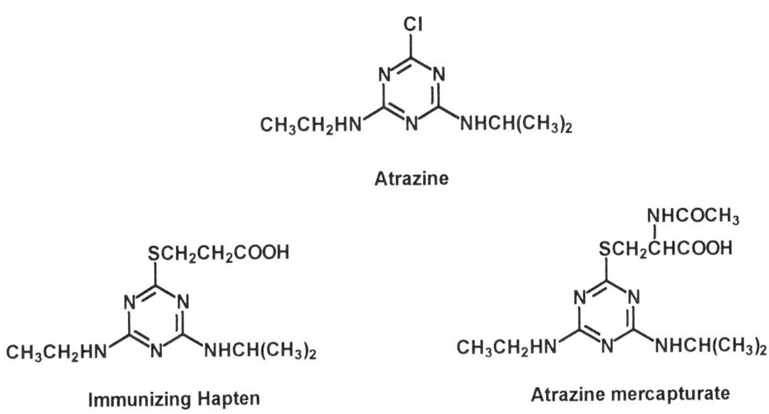


**Figure 6.** Structures of atrazine, the pesticide mimic used to raise antibodies recognizing atrazine and the N-acetylcysteine derivative of atrazine.

Through a series of classical extraction and partition methods, the immunoreactivity of the urine samples was followed. At no time did the material behave as the parent atrazine, or any of the N-dealkylated metabolites. Efforts to extract the urine sample and analyze by GC-MS for definitive confirmation were unsuccessful due to interfering co-extractants and problems involved with the formation and stability of GC derivatives of mercapturates. In order to circumvent this problem the antibody was used to extract the immunoreactive material. The antibody-extracted material was then analyzed by tandem mass spectrometry. The molecular weight and fragmentation pattern obtained for the antibody-extracted material matched exactly the spectrum for a synthesized standard of atrazine mercapturate (Lucas et al., 1993).

Attempts to analyze the mercapturate of atrazine by classical GC/MS techniques illustrate the exceptional difficulty of such an approach. The molecule contains a variety of polar functional groups that normally require derivatization for successful GC analysis. However, numerous derivatization schemes proved unsuccessful due to their instability under conditions of GC analysis. To complicate matters further, mercapturates co-extract with large amounts of endogenous compounds that share functionality and physical properties with mercapturates.

Alternate strategies such as HPLC analysis and direct probe MS suffer from interferences from the large mass of endogenous biological substances present in urine. In turn, affinity extraction with antibodies capable of binding to triazines was found to be the best approach for separating the mercapturate of atrazine from the complex urine matrix. By combining an affinity extraction system using a triazine selective antibody with FAB ionization tandem mass spectrometry, the presence of the mercapturate in urine was verified.

These same urine samples were then re-analyzed by immunoassay for atrazine mercapturate and by GC for the N-dealkylated metabolites. Table 3 shows the results of these analyses. Very little N-dealkylated metabolites were found in these samples. However, these metabolites were found in other sample sets analyzed soon after collection. Subsequently, we have found that these materials were not stable in urine samples under the storage conditions used. Thus, in these particular samples, these metabolites may have degraded. No further work has been conducted on this sample set. However, it is important to note that the mercapturate is still present in easily measured amounts. Thus, although this may not be the major metabolite present initially, it is certainly a more stable metabolite, present in large quantities and may thus be a useful biomarker of exposure. Subsequent studies have been conducted which describe this work in greater detail (Lucas et al., 1993).

These results indicate some of the properties of a compound that make it a good indicator of exposure in monitoring studies. First, of course, is abundance. The atrazine mercapturate is far more abundant in urine than the parent compound, thus increasing the limit of detection of exposure over 100 fold. A second attribute is analytical sensitivity. Although the immunoassays for the triazine herbicides are very sensitive, the larger size of the mercapturate makes the assay even more sensitive. Generality is a third attribute. The same mercapturate will be formed by a variety of different triazine herbicides with chloro, methoxy or thiomethyl in the 2- position thus making the assay selective for a variety of herbicides in this class (Figure 7). The antibody used also will detect mercapturates with varying R groups in the 4 and 6 positions making the triazine mercapturate a useful biomarker of exposure for the class of compounds. Since urine and other body fluids often are stored or transported before analysis, the apparent stability of the mercapturate relative to other possible biomarkers is a fourth attraction. In the case of atrazine, the presence of the mercapturate is a direct indication of the efficiency of glutathione conjugation, while with compounds like the S-methyl triazines, it is indicative of both sulfoxidation and conjugation. Thus, the biological relevance of the marker can be important. Of course, the ability to extrapolate from the urinary levels

**Table 3.** Concentration of metabolites in urine from volunteers exposed to atrazine

| Set No./ Sample No.[2] | Atrazine Mercapturate (ppb) | Metabolite 1[1] (ppb) | Metabolite 2 (ppb) |
|---|---|---|---|
| 1/1 | n.d.[3] | n.d. | n.d. |
| 1/2 | 234 | 16 | 26 |
| 1/3 | 493 | 70 | 5 |
| 1/4 | 131 | 7 | 7 |
| 1/5 | 18 | 1 | n.d |
| 2/1 | 377 | 18 | n.d. |
| 2/2 | 556 | 43 | n.d. |
| 2/3 | 58 | n.d. | 1 |
| 2/4 | 10 | n.d. | n.d. |
| 2/5 | 2 | n.d. | n.d. |

1 Metabolite 1 is the N-deethyl metabolite of atrazine. Metabolite 2 is the N-deisopropyl metabolite of atrazine.

2 Set and sample numbers correspond to the designations used in Figure 4. Sample number 6 in set 2 contained less than 1 ppb atrazine mercapturate and no detectable N-dealkylated metabolites.

3 n.d. = not detectable. Atrazine mercapturate was analyzed by ELISA. The limit of detectability was 0.1 ng/mL. N-dealkyl metabolites of atrazine were analyzed by GC. The limit of detectability was 1 ng/mL.

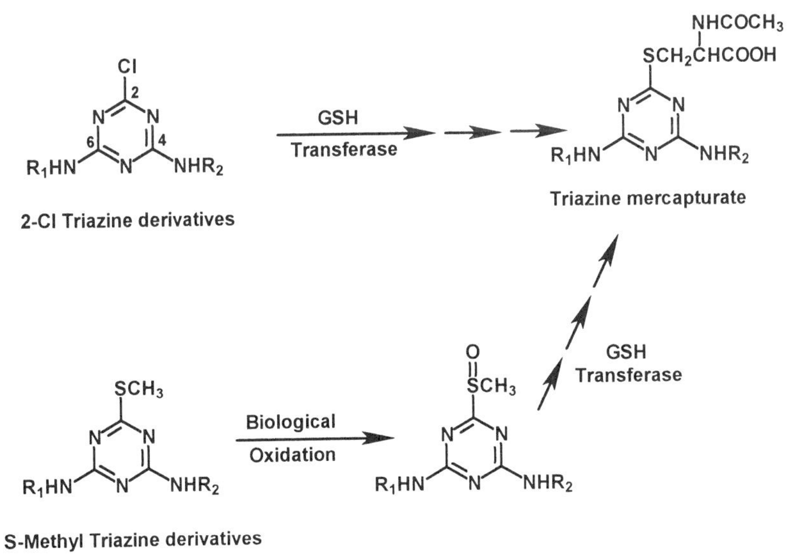


**Figure 7.** Proposed metabolic pathways to the N-acetylcysteine derivatives of triazines from the 2-chloro- (i.e., atrazine or simazine) and 2-thiomethyl triazines (i.e., ametryn or prometryn).

detected back to the amount of actual exposure is critical for many studies, and the data to support such an extrapolation are still lacking with the triazines.

## STATE OF THE TECHNOLOGY

Immunochemical methods have been demonstrated to be useful in the analysis of pesticides and pesticide metabolites. Up until fairly recently the development of this technology was somewhat limited to a few laboratories. Currently, however, there are companies that develop and manufacture test kits for a limited number of pesticides. Most immunoassay development appears to be occurring in-house in the various agrochemical companies. Regulatory agencies are moving toward acceptance of this technology and data generated by this technology. In general, immunoassay is being included among all analytical techniques. Guidelines for acceptance include such parameters as sensitivity, accuracy, precision, bias, matrix effects, and limit of detectability. Thus, we have seen over the past few years a movement toward integration of immunochemical techniques into the realm of environmental analytical chemistry. Due to the simplicity of conducting analyses and the potential for use in the field, immunochemical technology developers are concerned with standardization of test kits, proper use of the technology and appropriate interpretation of the resulting data. It is imperative that the user be aware of potential pitfalls of the technology, that proper quality control samples are run and that a good quality assurance program be in place. These are among the issues currently being addressed by a consortium of representatives from test kit manufacturers, the agrochemical industry, regulatory agencies and academia.

There are a number of interesting areas of research revolving around this technology. These include application to other compound types, such as chemicals commonly found at hazardous waste sites (i.e., dioxins (Stanker et al., 1987), nitroaromatic compounds (Eck et al., 1990) and metals (Wylie et al., 1991)), or exploring the limits of sensitivity (Schneider and Hammock, 1992). New applications for immunoassay also exist. For example immunoassays may be used as post-column detectors for HPLC (de Frutos and Regnier, 1993; Krämer et al., 1994), and have been used in antibody-based biosensors (Anis and Eldefrawi, 1993), and for sample cleanup (Trucksess et al., 1990). Experimentation is needed to make aspects of immunoassay development more predictive, and thus easier and quicker to develop. For example, addressing such problems as designing the best hapten to synthesize for a particular pesticide target, or determining which characteristics of the immunoreagents are most important for developing assays of desired sensitivity or selectivity. Finally, greater understanding is needed regarding the detector itself - the antibody. Molecular biology techniques allow us to potentially "engineer" antibody-binding to maximize or minimize binding as desired (Winter and Milstein, 1991).

## CONCLUSIONS

Due to the historical success of immunochemical techniques in clinical analysis, it seems likely that this technique is well suited for analysis of biomarkers of exposure to pesticides. One example of such an application has been described here for the triazine mercapturates. Immunoassay meets a variety of needs, from large sample throughput, through ability to conduct analyses "on-site" and low cost per analysis. As with any analytical method, however, understanding the principles of immunoassay and its strengths and weaknesses will provide more valid data generated by this method. Questions still exist as to who will develop, and implement immunoassays for general use and quality assurance issues must also be addressed. Nevertheless, it is certainly a technique that should be considered when designing exposure assessment studies.

## ACKNOWLEDGMENTS

The authors thank A. Dan Jones, Facility for Advanced Instrumentation, University of California at Davis for his helpful and timely review. This work was supported in part by NIEHS Superfund 2P42-ES04699, U.S. Environmental Protection Agency (EPA) Cooperative Research Grant CR819047, NIEHS Center for Environmental Health Sciences (at U.C. Davis) 1P30 ES05707; U.S. EPA. Center for Ecological Health Research at U.C. Davis CR819658 and U.S.D.A./P.S.W. 5-93-25 (Forest Service NAPIAP).

Although the information in this document has been funded in part by the United States Environmental Protection Agency, it may not necessarily reflect the views of the Agency and no official endorsement should be inferred.

## REFERENCES

Ames, B.N., Shigenaga, M.K., and Hagen, T.M., 1993, Oxidants, antioxidants, and the degenerative diseases of aging, *Proc. Natl. Acad. Sci. USA* 90:7915.

Anis, N.A., and Eldefrawi, M.E., 1993, Reusable fiber optic immunosensor for rapid detection of imazethapyr herbicide, *J. Agric. Food Chem.* 41:843.

Centeno, E.R., and Johnson, W.J., 1970, Antibodies to two common pesticides, DDT and malathion, *Int. Arch. Allergy Appl. Immunol.* 37:1.

Cheung, P.Y.K., and Hammock, B.D., 1988, Monitoring BT in the Environment with ELISA, *in:* "Biotechnology for Crop Protection," P.A. Hedin, J.J. Menn and R.M. Hollingworth, eds., American Chemical Society, Washington, DC.

de Frutos, M., and Regnier, F.E., 1993, Tandem chromatographic-immunological analyses, *Anal. Chem.* 65:17.

Dewey, M., Evans, D., Coleman, J., Priestley, R., Hull, R., Horsley, D., and Hawes, C., 1991, Antibodies in plant science, *Acta Bot. Neerl.* 40:1.

Eck, D.L., Kurth, M.J., and Macmillan, C., 1990, Trinitrotoluene and Other Nitroaromatic Compounds: Immunoassay Methods, *in:* "Immunochemical Methods for Environmental Analysis," J.M. Van Emon and R.O. Mumma, eds., American Chemical Society, Washington, D.C.

Engvall, E., and Perlmann, P., 1972, Enzyme-linked immunosorbent assay, ELISA. III. Quantitation of specific antibodies by enzyme-labeled anti-immunoglobulin in antigen-coated tubes, *J. Immunol.* 109:129.

Feng, P.C.C., Horton, S.R., and Sharp, C.R., 1992, A general method for developing immunoassays to chloroacetanilide herbicides, *J. Agric. Food Chem.* 40:211.

Gee, S.J., Hammock, B.D., and Van Emon, J.M., 1994, "A User's Guide to Environmental Immunochemical Analysis", Environmental Monitoring Systems Laboratory, U.S. Environmental Protection Agency, Las Vegas, NV 89109, EPA/540/R-94/509.

Gee, S.J., Miyamoto, T., Goodrow, M.H., Buster, D., and Hammock, B.D., 1988, Development of an enzyme-linked immunosorbent assay for the analysis of the thiocarbamate herbicide molinate, *J. Agric. Food Chem.* 36:863.

Goodrow, M.H., Harrison, R.O., and Hammock, B.D., 1990, Hapten synthesis, antibody development, and competitive inhibition enzyme immunoassay for s-triazine herbicides, *J. Agric. Food Chem.* 38:990.

Hall, J.C., Deschamps, R.J.A., and McDermott, M.R., 1990, Immunoassays to detect and quantitate herbicides in the environment, *Weed Technol.* 4:226.

Hammock, B.D., 1988, Applications of immunochemistry in crop protection and biotechnology, an overview, *in:* "Biotechnology for Crop Protection," P.A. Hedin, J.J. Menn and R.M. Hollingworth, eds., American Chemical Society, Washington, DC.

Hammock, B.D., and Mumma, R.O., 1980, Potential of immunochemical technology for pesticide analysis, *in:* "Recent Advances in Pesticide Analytical Methodology,"J. Harvey, Jr. and G. Zweig, eds., American Chemical Society, Washington, DC.

Harrison, R.O., Gee, S.J., and Hammock, B.D., 1988, Immunochemical methods of pesticide analysis, *in:* "Biotechnology for Crop Protection," P.A. Hedin, J.J. Menn and R.M. Hollingworth, eds., American Chemical Society, Washington, DC.

Harrison, R.O., Goodrow, M.H., and Hammock, B.D., 1991, Competitive inhibition ELISA for the s-triazine herbicides: Assay optimization and antibody characterization, *J. Agric. Food Chem.* 39:122.

Hayashi, Y., Shono, F., Yamamoto, S., Takasaki, W., Nakagawa, A., Watanabe, K., Yamashita, K., and Miyazaki, H., 1990, Immunoaffinity purification of 11-dehydro-thromboxane B2 from human urine and plasma for quantitative analysis by radioimmunoassay, *Anal. Biochem.* 187:151.

Jung, F., Gee, S.J., Harrison, R.O., Goodrow, M.H., Karu, A.E., Braun, A.L., Li, Q.X., and Hammock, B.D., 1989, Use of immunochemical techniques for the analysis of pesticides, *Pest. Sci.* 26:303.

Karu, A.E., Harrison, R.O., Schmidt, D.J., Clarkson, C.E., Grassman, J., Goodrow, M.H., Lucas, A., Hammock, B.D., Van Emon, J.M., and White, R.J., 1991, Monoclonal immunoassay of triazine herbicides: development and implementation, *in:* "Immunoassays for Trace Chemical Analysis: Monitoring Toxic Chemicals in Humans, Food, and the Environment.," M. Vanderlaan, L.H. Stanker, B.E. Watkins and D.W. Roberts, eds., American Chemical Society, Washington, DC.

Katz, S.E., and Brady, M.S., 1990, High performance immunoaffinity chromatography for drug residue analysis, *J. Assoc. Off. Anal. Chem.* 73:557.

Krämer, P.M., Li, Q.X., and Hammock, B.D., 1993, Integration of LC with immunoassay: an approach combining the potential of both methods, *J. A.O.A.C. Int.,* 77:1275.

Landsteiner, K., 1945, "The Specificity of Serological Reactions," Harvard University Press, Cambridge, Massachusetts.

Langone, J.J., and van Vunakis, H., 1975, Radioimmunoassay for dieldrin and aldrin, *Res. Commun. Chem. Pathol. Pharmacol.* 10:163.

Lawruk, T.S., Lachman, C.E., Jourdan, S.W., Fleeker, J.R., Herzog, D.P., and Rubio, F.M., 1993, Determination of metolachlor in water and soil by a rapid magnetic particle-based ELISA, *J. Agric. Food Chem.* 41:1426.

Lee, L.S., Wall, J.H., Cotty, P.J., and Bayman, P., 1990, Integration of enzyme-linked immunosorbent assay with conventional chromatographic procedures for quantitation of aflatoxin in individual cotton bolls, seeds, and seed sections, *J. Assoc. Off. Anal. Chem.* 73:581.

Li, Q., Zhao, M., Gee, S.J., Kurth, M., Seiber, J.N., and Hammock, B.D., 1991, Development of enzyme-linked immunosorbent assays for 4-nitrophenol and substituted 4-nitrophenols, *J. Agric. Food Chem.* 39:1685.

Lucas, A.D., Jones, A.D., Goodrow, M.H., Saiz, S.G., Blewett, C., Seiber, J.N., and Hammock, B.D., 1993, Determination of atrazine metabolites in human urine: Development of a biomarker of exposure, *Chem. Res. Toxicol.* 6:107.

Lucas, A.D., Schneider, P., Harrison, R.O., Seiber, J.N., Hammock, B.D., Biggar, J.W., and Rolston, D.E., 1992, Determination of atrazine and simazine in water and oil using polyclonal and monoclonal antibodies in enzyme-linked immunosorbent assays, *Food Agric. Immunol.* 3:155.

Marco, M.-P., Gee, S.J., Cheng, H.M., Liang, Z.Y., and Hammock, B.D., 1993, Development of an enzyme-linked immunosorbent assay for carbaryl, *J. Agric. Food Chem.* 41:423.

McDiarmid, M.A., and Strickland, P.T., 1990, DNA adducts as markers of exposure in hazardous waste workers, *Occ. Med.* 5:49.

Rodbard, D., 1981, Mathematics and statistics of ligand assays: an illustrated guide, *in:* "Ligand Assay: Analysis of International Developments on Isotopic and Nonisotopic Immunoassay," J. Langan and J.J. Clapp, eds., Masson Publishing USA, Inc., New York.

Schlaeppi, J., Meyer, W., and Ramsteiner, K.A., 1992, Determination of triasulfuron in soil by monoclonal antibody-based enzyme immunoassay, *J. Agric. Food Chem.* 40:1093.

Schneider, P., and Hammock, B.D., 1992, Influence of the ELISA format and the hapten-enzyme conjugate on the sensitivity of an immunoassay for s-triazine herbicides using monoclonal antibodies, *J. Agric. Food Chem.* 40:525.

Skerritt, J.H., Hill, A.S., Beasley, H.L., Edward, S.L., and McAdam, D.P., 1992, Enzyme-linked immunosorbent assay for quantitation of organophosphate pesticides: fenitrothion, chlorpyrifos-methyl, and pirimiphos-methyl in wheat grain and flour-milling fractions, *J. A.O.A.C. Int.* 75:519.

Stanker, L.H., Bigbee, C., Van Emon, J., Watkins, B., Jense, R.H., Morris, C., and Vanderlaan, M., 1989, An immunoassay for pyrethroids: Detection of permethrin in meat, *J. Agric. Food Chem.* 37:834.

Stanker, L.H., Watkins, B., Rogers, N., and Vanderlaan, M., 1987, Monoclonal antibodies for dioxin: antibody characterization and assay development, *Toxicol.* 45:229.

Tijssen, P., 1985, "Practice and Theory of Enzyme Immunoassays," Elsevier, Amsterdam.

Trucksess, M.W., Young, K., Donahue, K.F., Morris, D.K. and Lewis, E., 1990, Comparison of two immunochemical methods with thin-layer chromatographic methods for determination of aflatoxins, *J. Assoc. Off. Anal. Chem.* 73:425.

Van Emon, J., Hammock, B., and Seiber, J.N., 1986, Enzyme-linked immunosorbant assay for paraquat and its application to exposure analysis, *Anal. Chem.* 58:1866.

Van Emon, J.M., and Lopez-Avila, V., 1992, Immunochemical methods for environmental analysis, *Anal. Chem.* 64:79.

Voller, A., Bidwell, D.E., and Bartlett, A., 1976, Enzyme immunoassay in diagnostic medicine. Theory and practice, *Bull. World Health Organ.* 53:55.

Wie, S.I., and Hammock, B.D., 1984, Comparison of coating and immunizing antigen structure on the sensitivity and specificity of immunoassays for benzoylphenylurea insecticides, *J. Agric. Food Chem.* 32:1294.

Wing, K.D., Hammock, B.D., and Wustner, D.A., 1978, Development of an S-bioallethrin specific antibody, *J. Agric. Food Chem.* 26:1328.

Winter, G., and Milstein, C., 1991, Man-made antibodies, *Nature* 349:293.

Wittmann, C., and Hock, B., 1993, Analysis of atrazine residues in food by an enzyme immunoassay, *J. Agric. Food Chem.* 41:1421.

Wong, R.B., and Ahmed, Z.H., 1992, Development of an enzyme-linked immunosorbent assay for imazaquin herbicide, *J. Agric. Food Chem.* 40:811.

Wylie, D.E., Carlson, L.D., Carlson, R., Wagner, F.W., and Schuster, S.M., 1991, Detection of mercuric ions in water by ELISA with a mercury-specific antibody, *Anal. Biochem.* 194:381.

Yalow, R.S., and Berson, S.A., 1959, Radiobiology: Assay of plasma insulin human subjects by immunological methods, *Nature* 184:1648.

Yalow, R.S., and Berson, S.A., 1960, Immunoassay of endogenous plasma insulin in man, *J. Clin. Invest.* 39:1157.

# THE USE OF BIOMARKERS IN THE EPIDEMIOLOGICAL SURVEILLANCE OF PESTICIDE WORKERS

Antonella Fait[1] and Marco Maroni[2]

[1]International Centre for Pesticide Safety
Via Magenta 25 - 20020 Busto Garolfo (Milano) - Italy

[2]Institute of Occupational Medicine
University of Milan
Via S. Barnaba 8 - 20100 Milano - Italy

In this paper we address some issues related to the practical use of "biomarkers" for the epidemiological surveillance of workers occupationally exposed to pesticides, either in industrial or agricultural settings.

## EPIDEMIOLOGICAL EVALUATION OF HEALTH EFFECTS FROM PROLONGED EXPOSURE TO PESTICIDES

At the International Centre for Pesticide Safety, we have recently reviewed the epidemiological studies on long-term health effects from pesticides published over the last 20 years[1]. Despite the remarkable number of investigations (we have collected more than 400 papers), very few studies present requisites which allow clear demonstrations or causal inference to be made. The main problems in the design of epidemiological studies on pesticide-exposed workers relate to the difficulty in accurately estimating and quantifying exposure. Secondly, investigated long-term health effects are not specific, occur after a long latency period, and often belong to the group of "rare event" outcomes.

In many cases information on the type of pesticides handled is lacking, especially in studies on agricultural workers. Multiple exposure to mixtures of compounds or concomitant exposure to contaminants, intermediates of production and other risk factors often occur. Exposure assessment commonly relies on job classification and estimates of pesticide exposures reported to be associated with these jobs. Job classification is based on interviews in case-control studies, and on employment records or death certificates in cohort studies. Surrogate measures of exposure, such as types of crops or number of acres sprayed, are often used to characterize exposure of agricultural workers. Only in a minority of studies environmental or biological monitoring data are available.

The traditional epidemiological approach to the health-risk assessment of human

*Methods of Pesticide Exposure Assessment*, Edited by
P.B. Curry *et al.*, Plenum Press, New York, 1995

exposure to pesticides has produced little "strong" information: as shown in the table which concluded our review (Table 1), this approach has been successful in finding associations and establishing causality only for a few outcomes, while most of the reported observations remain vague and difficult to prove.

## RATIONALE FOR THE USE OF BIOMARKERS IN EXPOSURE ASSESSMENT

The application of biomarkers in studies of occupational exposure to hazardous chemicals is now recognized as a useful tool to improve the effectiveness of epidemiological surveillance [2, 4, 5]. In particular, the use of biomarkers to improve documentation of exposure is a crucial point, because misclassification of individual exposures reduces the power of studies to detect health effects, and may produce misleading results. Exposure misclassification tends to reduce estimates of relative risk and to dilute exposure-response gradients [6]. Biomarkers improve specificity and sensitivity of exposure measurements, and therefore reduce the potential for exposure misclassification.

The incorporation of exposure markers in epidemiological studies of pesticide workers can supplement traditional methods of exposure evaluation, thus enabling researchers to overcome many of the difficulties mentioned above. Biomarkers provide in fact the best opportunity to:

1. Confirm the nature of exposure and gather accurate information on the type of pesticides absorbed. This is of extreme value especially in studies on pesticide applicators and agricultural workers, who are typically exposed to many different compounds, either simultaneously or successively;
2. Provide measurements of internal dose, that is of the amount of pesticide or of its metabolites, absorbed through all possible routes and, in some cases, over the entire period of exposure. This is particularly suitable for the assessment of exposure to pesticides, because of the various routes of exposure involved and of the possible combination of occupational and nonoccupational exposures. This is also important when considering that dose estimates provided by air monitoring, which has more often been measured historically than biologic concentrations, give an indication of doses received by inhalation, which are of limited relevance for pesticides, since skin is the most significant route of absorption for most compounds;
3. Provide measurements of the biological effective dose, which indicates the amount of pesticide that has interacted with critical subcellular targets. For instance, the determination of DNA or Hb pesticide adducts, provide measurement of the dose of compound which has formed stable covalent bonds with cellular macromolecules.

## CONSTRAINTS OF THE USE OF BIOMARKERS IN SURVEILLANCE PROGRAMMES

In spite of these advantages, so far biomarkers have not been frequently applied to surveillance programmes of workers exposed to pesticides. One of the main reasons for the limited application of biomarkers relates to the availability of indicators. There are more than 700 active compounds incorporated in approximately 10,000 different formulations; however, biological monitoring indices have been tested for about one tenth.

For some pesticides currently in use biomarkers have been studied only in experimental systems, and have still to be validated in man.

**Table 1.** Reported health effects from prolonged exposure to pesticides

| Pesticide/Classes | Further confirmation required | Well-documented evidence |
|---|---|---|
| Phenoxy herbicides:<br>2,4,5-T<br>2,4-D<br>MCPA<br>contaminants (TCDD TCPA) | Soft-tissue sarcoma<br>Lymphomas, Leukemias<br>Stomach cancer<br>Colon cancer<br>Prostate cancer<br>Teratogenetic effects | Chloracne (TCDD) |
| Other herbicides:<br>Triazines<br>Arsenicals | Ovarian cancer | Lung cancer<br>Liver diseases |
| Halogenated hydrocarbons:<br>1,3-Dichloropropene<br>PCP<br>DBCP<br>Methylbromide<br>EDB | Lymphomas, Leukemias<br>Aplastic anemia<br>Neurotoxic effects | Spermatogenesis suppression<br>Sperm abnormalities |
| Carbamates:<br>Carbaryl | Chromosome aberrations<br>Sperm abnormalities | |
| Organochlorines:<br>Chlordane/Heptachlor<br>Hexachlorobenzene<br>DDT | Blood dyscrasias<br>Brain cancer<br>Liver cancer<br>Chromosome aberrations<br>High cholesterol/triglycerides<br>Tremors, muscular weakness | Porphyria<br>Chloracne |
| Pyrethroids: | | Paresthesias |
| Organophosphates: | Chromosome aberrations<br>SNC effects<br>Lymphomas | Delayed neuropathy[1] |
| Copper Sulfate: | Liver diseases | |

[1] Some compounds only, after subacute or acute exposure.

For some biological indicators related to chemical contaminants that are ubiquitous in the environment, definition of reference values in the population and assessment of other routes of exposure (for instance diet) is necessary for the correct interpretation of biological monitoring results. In the use of biomarkers, knowledge about intra- and inter-individual variability in the population is essential. For the most recent indicators, such as DNA or protein adducts, such information is generally not available.

Technical issues related to analytical complexity, difficulties in preserving or transporting the samples, and high costs of laboratory measurements also represent major limits for the application of biomarkers to large groups of subjects.

Finally, constraints related to invasiveness of the procedures play a role as well. Sampling of adipose tissue for the evaluation of exposure to lipid-soluble compounds (such as the organochlorine DDT) for instance, provides excellent information on the dose of compound which accumulates in the body, but this procedure may be questioned if it requires a surgical action.

Markers such as chromosome aberrations or DNA adducts, which involve mutagenic effects, may be related to the formation of cancers, even though their real significance is not completely understood; in these cases the question of how to treat this information with the individual subject is not simple to be answered and might pose ethical difficulties to the practical use of these indicators.

## BIOMARKERS OF EXPOSURE TO PESTICIDES

Table 2 shows an overview of conventional biomarkers for biological monitoring of human exposure to various pesticides [7, 8, 3]. The reported tests include two types of measurements: a) unchanged pesticides or their metabolites in urine or blood, and b) measurements of biological effect of the pesticides, such as red blood cell acetylcholinesterase activity in individuals exposed to organophosphorous compounds.

It should be noted that for some compounds, such as for example the substituted urea herbicides (linuron, monuron), biological monitoring tests for routine use have not been developed. For other compounds, for example organotins, uncertainties still exist. Blood and urine concentrations of tin have been proposed as biomarkers to confirm exposure to organotin compounds; but since tin is commonly found also in nonexposed individuals with wide interindividual variations, in the absence of baseline reference values prior to exposure, the interpretation of the biological meaning of this indicator is difficult.

In addition to these conventional indicators a new generation of biomarkers is currently under development. Protein and DNA adducts have been detected for a variety of pesticides. Table 3, for example, shows a list of pesticides which form protein conjugates in erythrocytes. A dose-dependent relationship between haemoglobin adducts and exposure has been reported in the literature for pesticides of different chemical classes. The chemicals need to be converted into reactive metabolites in order to form adducts; therefore, the measurement of specific protein adducts provides an integrated information which also takes into account the ability of the organism to form reactive metabolites and to generate a biological effective dose. Thus adduct formation allows a better estimate of the biological risk. Due to the stability of the linkage to proteins, these markers also provide opportunity for integrating exposures which fluctuate over time.

## THE EPIDEMIOLOGICAL SURVEILLANCE PROGRAMME OF PESTICIDE WORKERS IN THE REGION OF LOMBARDY

A major problem is to decide when and how biological markers can be used for epidemiological surveillance. An accurate evaluation of the pattern and characteristics

**Table 2.** Biomarkers of exposure to pesticides

| Pesticides | Biomarkers | Blood | Urine |
|---|---|---|---|
| ORGANOPHOSPHATES | AChe, PChe | + | |
| | Alkylphosphates | | + |
| | Compound/metabolites | + | + |
| CARBAMATES | AChe, PChe | + | |
| carbaryl | α-naphtol | + | + |
| propoxur | 2-isopropoxyphenol | | + |
| DITHIOCARBAMATES | Compound/metabolites | + | + |
| | $CS_2$ | | + |
| EBDC | ETU | | + |
| PYRETHROIDS | | | |
| permethrin | $Cl_2CA$ | | + |
| deltamethrin | $Br_2CA$ | | + |
| | deltamethrin | | + |
| fenvalerate | fenvalerate | | + |
| ORGANOCHLORINES | Compound/metabolites | + | + |
| dieldrin, aldrin | dieldrin | + | |
| lindane | lindane | + | + |
| endrin | anti-12 hydroxyendrin | | + |
| DDT | DDT | + | |
| TRIAZINES | | | |
| atrazine | atrazine | | + |
| | dealkylated atrazine | | + |
| s-triazines | cyanuric acid | | + |
| SUBSTITUTED UREAS | not available | | |
| flufenoxuron | flufenoxuron | + | |
| ORGANOTIN COMPOUNDS | not available | | |
| | tin (?) | + | + |
| MORPHOLINES | not available | | |
| trifenmorph | morpholine | | + |
| | triphenylcarbinol | | + |
| PHENOXYACETATES | | | |
| 2,4-D | 2,4-D | | + |
| MCPA | MCPA | | + |
| OTHERS | | | |
| diquat | diquat | + | + |
| paraquat | paraquat | + | + |
| chlordimeform | 4-COT | | + |
| carbamate herbicides/ fungicides | not available | | |

of exposure is required before applying biomarkers to surveillance programmes. How this can be carried out will be illustrated with the example of a programme for the epidemiological surveillance of pesticide workers which is currently under development in Lombardy.

The Region of Lombardy, located in the North of Italy, covers an area of approximately 24,000 squared kilometres, with a population of about nine millions. The cultivated agricultural area accounts for approximately 50% of the total area, with about

**Table 3.** Pesticides which form protein conjugates in erythrocytes

| | |
|---|---|
| Amitrole | Metamitron |
| Anilazine | Methiocarb |
| Azocyclotin | p-Nitrophenol |
| Carbofuran | Omethoate |
| Chlordimeform | Phoxim |
| Demeton-S-methyl | Propanil |
| Diuron | Propineb |
| Fenfluthrin | Propoxur |
| Fuberidazole | Triadimefon |

200,000 subjects employed in agricultural work. In this area the International Centre for Pesticide Safety, on behalf of the Regional Public Health Authority, is establishing an epidemiological observatory which, among other purposes, will allow to perform specific epidemiological investigations on selected subgroups of the farming population and on workers employed in the manufacture of pesticides.

The programme is composed of several subsequent phases. First of all, based on available census data on land use, farms, and cultivations, subgroups of workers employed in specific settings and characterized by homogeneous exposure patterns (for instance, manufacturers of specific compounds, professional sprayers, greenhouse workers, wine growers, rice growers, etc.) are identified. Systematic and accurate collection of data on type of pesticides used, amounts, and days of application or of exposure are set up, and exposure modelling is performed on the basis of the collected data. The use of biomarkers will then be applied only to selected groups, for which specific exposures can be well defined and documented, in order to validate exposure modelling. Exposure registries of workers in pesticide manufacture and application are thus established for a long-term individual follow-up.

Once exposure registries are available, cohort studies can be planned to monitor the occurrence of specific health outcomes of interest. For instance, an objective could be to evaluate the association between exposure to pesticides and the occurrence of reproductive effects, in particular congenital malformations. The occurrence of long-term health outcomes, cancer and noncancer effects, can also be studied within identified cohorts from registered subjects. However, in this case the long latency will make the registries established today usable only in the future, after two or three decades.

It should be noted that this surveillance programme entails the collection of an enormous amount of data. Such collection of data is made possible in our case by the existence of an extended territorial network of public occupational health units: 84 Local Health Units with a professional team, 8 Hospital Departments and 14 Multizone Laboratories will cooperate for the creation of this database and for the epidemiological surveillance of pesticide workers.

In conclusion, we believe that use of biomarkers in epidemiological surveillance is necessary and extremely promising. However, to overcome the serious practical problems connected with their use, comprehensive public health programmes have to be created and implemented.

This work has been in part supported by the National Research Council of Italy (Targeted Project "Prevention and Control Disease Factors" FATMA-SP2, grant n.93.00688.PF41).

## REFERENCES

1. Maroni, M., and Fait, A., "Health Effects in Man from Long-term Exposure to Pesticides. A Review of the 1975-1991 Literature", *Toxicol.* 78, Elsevier Scientific Publishers, Ireland (1993).
2. Hulka, B.S., Wilkosky, T.C., and Griffith, J.D., "Biological Markers in Epidemiology", Oxford University Press, New York (1990).
3. Brewster, M.A., Hulka, B.S., and Lavy, T.L., Biomarkers of pesticide exposure, *Rev. Environ. Contam. Toxicol.* 128:17-42 (1992).
4. Griffith, J.D., Duncan, R., and Hulka, B.S., Biochemical and biological markers: implications for epidemiologic studies, *Arch. Environ. Health.* 44(6):375-381 (1989).
5. Hulka, B.S., and Wilkosky, T.C., Biological markers in epidemiologic research, *Arch. Environ. Health.* 43(2):83-93 (1988).
6. Blair, A., Hoar Zham, S., Cantor., K.P., and Stewart, P.A., Estimating exposure to pesticides in epidemiological studies of cancer, *in*: "Biological Monitoring for Pesticide Exposure. Measurement, Estimation, and Risk Reduction", R.G.M. Wang, C.A. Franklin, R.C. Honeycutt, and J.C. Reinert, eds., ACS Symp. Series 382:38-46, American Chemical Society, Washington, D.C. (1989).
7. He, F., Biological monitoring of occupational pesticide exposure, *Int. Arch. Occup. Environ. Health.* 65:S69-S76 (1993).
8. Tordoir, W.F., Maroni, M., and He. F., "Health Surveillance of Pesticide Workers. A Manual for Occupational Health Professionals", *Toxicol.* 91, Elsevier Scientific Publishers, Ireland (1994).

# BIOMARKER TESTING FOR THE ASSESSMENT OF POPULATIONS EXPOSED TO HAZARDOUS CHEMICALS

Michael Straight*

Formerly with (ATSDR)
Allergy Respiratory Institute of Colorado
5800 East Evans Ave.
Denver, CO 80222

Robert W. Amler

United States Public Health Service
Agency for Toxic Substances and Disease Registry
Atlanta, GA 30333

Robert F. Vogt

Division of Environmental Health Laboratory Sciences
Centers for Disease Control
Atlanta, GA 30333

Howard M. Kipen

Environmental and Occupational Health Sciences Institute
RW Johnson Medical School
Piscataway, NJ 08855

## INTRODUCTION

A major challenge facing environmental scientists is to accurately document human exposure to hazardous substances and evaluate adverse human health effects which may result from such exposure. Current knowledge in this area suggests that adverse human health effects may be associated with chronic low dose exposure to hazardous substances. These effects can manifest as subclinical organ-system changes that may be detected prior to overt signs and symptoms of disease.

*Formerly with Division of Health Studies, Agency for Toxic Substances and Disease Registry

*Methods of Pesticide Exposure Assessment*, Edited by
P.B. Curry *et al.*, Plenum Press, New York, 1995

Health provisions of the Comprehensive Environmental Response, Compensation, and Liability Act of 1980 (CERCLA) mandate that the U.S. Public Health Service, specifically the Agency for Toxic Substances and Disease Registry (ATSDR), sponsor or conduct health studies of persons exposed to hazardous substances. Equally important is the increased concern expressed by citizens who live near NPL sites about potential adverse health effects which may result from exposure to hazardous substances. In responding to the legislative directive of CERCLA and growing citizen concern about possible adverse health effects related to exposure to hazardous substances, the Division of Health Studies of ATSDR has developed and used medical test batteries in its health studies. These test batteries are used to detect subclinical organ-system dysfunction in people who live near National Priority List (NPL) hazardous waste sites and to develop effective measures to mitigate possible adverse health effects. Population based studies will use established epidemiological and statistical methods to determine associations between environmental exposures and sub-clinical organ-system changes which may indicate disease. This talk outlines the approach and some of the challenges yet to be addressed as the Division of Health Studies undertakes activities in the relatively new and uncertain area of epidemiologic environmental exposure investigation.

## DEFINITION

The term "biomarker" has been used, in general, to mean a signal or indicator that serves as a guide or sets a boundary[1]. A biomarker could therefore refer to any indicator of the state of a biologic system. The National Research Council states that "... the concentration or presence of these markers represents points on a continuum. Therefore, the boundaries between health and disease may change as knowledge increases."[2] Biomarkers are used in an effort to predict the occurrence of adverse health effects, and perhaps allow preventive measures to be taken that would mitigate the health effects due to exposure to environmental toxicants.

For human environmental health studies, a biomarker of organ damage or dysfunction is defined as a measurable alteration in cells or cell products caused by an abnormal effect on a particular organ system. The alteration may be an increase or decrease in something that occurs normally (e.g., blood glucose), the presence of something not normally found (e.g., a toxicant or a metabolite, blood or protein in urine), or a change in the distribution of molecular species or cells (e.g., shifts in lymphocyte sub-populations). The accuracy and precision of the methods used to detect changes in biomarkers requires further development, as well as knowledge of the eventual long term health effects in the population studied so that predictive value of the biomarker can be determined.

Toxic exposure is one of the possible causes for abnormal biomarker test results, but there are many reasons why an organ system departs from homeostasis. Malignancy, pregnancy, infection, trauma, malnutrition, errors of metabolism, and physiologic stress can also cause biomarker changes and confound population studies. The use of comparison populations, questionnaires, analytical measurements of specific toxicants, and longitudinal followup of exposed populations are needed to determine whether the presence of a biomarker truly reflects the effects of toxic exposure and predicts future health effects.

Biomarkers can be used to identify: 1) susceptibility to the toxic effects of environmental pollutants; 2) exposure to such toxicants; and 3) biologic effects of exposure[3]. Susceptibility markers are measurable indicators of biologic factors that influence the probability of disease. Exposure markers are measurable indicators that can occur after the body is exposed to toxicant(s). The most obvious example of an exposure marker is the measured level of a toxicant in an organism. A biomarker of effect, measured usually in blood or urine, reflects change in an organ resulting from toxic effects, if other causes for the change are ruled out.

## BIOMARKER USE IN ENVIRONMENTAL HEALTH STUDIES

Why use biomarkers to assess populations? The lessons learned from previous exposure studies and symptom and disease prevalence studies of persons living near hazardous waste sites showed the need for better ways to segregate populations into those truly exposed and those unaffected. The typical population living near a hazardous waste site is exposed to low levels of several toxicants over many years via several pathways.

Vietnam veterans exposed to Agent Orange were classified into groups based on a historical ranking of exposure from interviews and Army personnel and environmental (spraying) records. The Vietnam ground troops study measured serum dioxin levels in these men many years later, and no correlation between the exposure classification of the participants and their serum dioxin levels was found. This study provides an illustration of the need for objective measures that reflect human exposure, as opposed to relying on the development of risk assessments for an exposed population that rely on exposure reconstruction or environmental toxicant levels.

## APPLICATION OF BIOMARKERS IN PUBLIC HEALTH

ATSDR is one of the lead federal agencies investigating the effect of environmental toxicants upon human populations. The exposures studied are chronic, low-level, and involve diverse pathways.

ATSDR commissioned the Board on Environmental Studies and Toxicology, National Research Council to publish a series of reports on biomarker testing, including Biologic Markers in Pulmonary Toxicology (1989), Biologic Markers in Reproductive Toxicology (1989), Biologic Markers in Immunotoxicology (1992), and Environmental Neurotoxicology (1992).

In the Neurotoxicology report, the committee hypothesized, based on the available evidence, that an as-yet-unspecified fraction of human neurologic and psychiatric disease is attributable to chemical agents in the environment. The committee recommended that a more accurate estimate of the extent of the problem of neurologic and psychiatric dysfunction attributable to chemical agents in the environment be made. The estimate must be based on a combination of clinical, epidemiologic, and toxicologic studies coupled with the techniques of quantitative risk assessment.

What evidence supports the estimate of the committee that neurotoxins may be a problem for the general population? Cross-sectional studies of populations exposed to hazardous chemical waste have occasionally found an increased odds ratio for neurologic disease and symptoms. One such study, in 1990, compared 713 persons living near a hazardous waste incinerator with 588 controls, and found statistically significantly increased odds ratios for neurologic signs and symptoms in the exposed population[4]. Since several studies suggested an increased prevalence of neurologic, pulmonary, and other organ system disease and symptoms, the problem facing ATSDR was how to test human populations objectively for the effects of exposure to hazardous chemicals found in the environment?

## PRIORITY HEALTH CONDITIONS

To address these needs for objective test methods, ATSDR began a project to develop the capacity to use biomarker testing in the assessment of populations exposed or potentially exposed to hazardous chemicals. To focus this effort, ATSDR reviewed adverse health outcomes potentially related to environmental exposure to toxic substances at hazardous waste sites. Seven priority health conditions were selected as broad categories of diseases, disorders, or dysfunctions for which human health studies and chemical-specific research are needed. These seven were selected based upon (1) the frequency of occurrence of adverse human health conditions at hazardous waste sites, (2) the severity of the adverse human health conditions associated with the substances selected, (3) the frequency or extent of concern expressed to physicians and public health practitioners by persons living near hazardous waste sites, and (4) the ability to prevent or mitigate the potentially causative exposures through medical care or prevention activities.

**Table 1.** ATSDR priority health conditions (in alphabetical order) for national environmental epidemiologic research efforts, United States, 1992

| |
|---|
| • Birth Defects and Reproductive Disorders |
| • Cancer (selected anatomic sites) |
| • Immune Function Disorders |
| • Kidney Dysfunction |
| • Liver Dysfunction |
| • Lung and Respiratory Diseases |
| • Neurotoxic Disorders |

Source: MMWR 1992 and ATSDR Priority Health Conditions[5]

In addition to selecting the priority health conditions, ATSDR identified the following four areas to further direct investigation activities:

- Evaluations of the occurrence of adverse health effects in specific populations.
- Identification of risk factors for adverse health effects from exposure to hazardous waste sites.
- Development of methods to diagnose adverse health effects.
- Diagnosis of adverse health effects in persons.

ATSDR is charged with implementing studies and research to address the priority health conditions and the concomitant four areas for investigation.

## MEDICAL TEST BATTERIES

A standard battery of medical tests for each of the seven priority health conditions has been proposed for use in ATSDR's health research program as biologic markers (biomarkers) of subclinical and clinical effects in several major organ systems, including effects on the immune system. Although not yet fully validated for population-based investigations, many of the proposed tests are commonly used by health care providers and health researchers for diagnosis and evaluation, and in concert with a history and physical examination and other diagnostic modalities can help detect early dysfunction of their respective organ systems.

Biomarker panels available in 1993 for the assessment of organ system function of human populations living near hazardous waste sites include:

a. Renal
b. Hepatobiliary
c. Immune
d. Pulmonary
e. Neurobehavioral
f. Reproductive (unpublished, available 1994)

To examine the prevalence of organ system function disorders, ATSDR is using these biomarker panels to select fieldworthy tests and conduct epidemiologic studies on exposed and reference populations. More definitive studies may then be designed for those organ system function disorders that are identified using the screening biomarker test panels. The use of these tests by ATSDR in multisite studies is intended to enhance statistical power by combining data from several study populations at comparable types of hazardous waste sites or other polluted geographic areas. For example, in 1991 and 1992, ATSDR interviewed and conducted medical test batteries, including immune testing, for nearly 3,000 study participants in 5 states, as part of a multisite exposure study.

A tier approach for biomarker testing at hazardous waste sites has been developed and endorsed by participants in workshops conducted by ATSDR to discuss the biomarker test panels. The tiers include a basic test battery, a reflex or focused test battery, and a research test battery. The basic test battery is the only tier that has been used thus far in the investigation of persons potentially exposed to hazardous waste by ATSDR.

Biomarker test batteries have not yet been used in the investigation of populations exposed primarily to pesticides. The neurobehavioral and immune test batteries would be the most likely to be used to evaluate a population exposed to pesticides. Therefore these will be discussed briefly.

The principal three classes of response seen in disease states affecting the immune system are hypersensitivity, immune deficiency, and autoimmunity. Such responses can occur due to adverse reactions to prescription medications, occupational exposures, or in some cases exposure to environmental toxicants. Much less is known about effects on the immune system that may result from exposure to environmental toxicants at low levels, such as those commonly found at hazardous waste site releases. However, certain classes of immune function disorders (for example, hypersensitivity) are usually not dose-related and may be triggered by extremely small quantities of foreign material[6].

The following features of immune tissues make them particularly susceptible to toxicant effects: (1) the rapid turnover of the cellular component, (2) the intricate control mechanisms required for effective host defense, (3) the inherent surveillance function of the immune system to react to foreign substances. In short, the basic function of the immune system, which is to recognize and neutralize substances identified as foreign, increases the likelihood of its exposure to systemically distributed toxicants.

Environmental toxicants have the potential for causing immunotoxic effects occurring after short- or long-term exposures, and may not be apparent until after a long latent period. In 1989, ATSDR published the Priority List of Hazardous Substances. This document, a CERCLA-mandated priority listing of hazardous substances, based on each substance's frequency of occurrence at NPL sites, toxicity, and potential for human exposure, was revised in 1992[7]. Of the 50 chemical substances ranked highest on the Priority List of 275 Hazardous Substances 30 are associated with adverse effects on the immune system. In addition, of the 10 most frequently identified substances at proposed or final NPL sites, 9 were known immunotoxicants based on the ATSDR hazardous

**Table 2.** Some compounds and substances that have been associated with immune effects in animals and/or humans, with emphasis on those occurring in occupational and hazardous waste settings

| Compound | Hypersensitivity | Immune Deficiency | Autoimmunity |
|---|---|---|---|
| Aluminum chloride | + | | |
| Arsenic | + | | |
| Asbestos | | + | |
| Benzene | | + | |
| Benzidine | | + | |
| 2-Butanone | + | ? | |
| Beryllium | + | | |
| Cadmium | + | + | + |
| Carbamates * | | + | |
| Chlorodibenzofurans | | + | |
| Chromium | + | | |
| Cobalt, metal fume and dust | + | | |
| Copper | + | + | |
| 2,4-dichlorophenol | | ? | |
| 1,3-dichloropropene | + | | |
| Dieldrin | | + | + |
| Formaldehyde | + | | |
| Hexachlorocyclohexane | + | | |
| Isocyanates | + | | |
| Lead | | + | |
| Methyl parathion | | + | |
| Mercury | + | + | ? |
| Nickel | + | | |
| Nitrosamines * | | ? | |
| Ozone * | ? | + | |
| Platinum salts * | + | | |
| Polychlorinated biphenyls and dioxins | + | + | |
| Polycyclic aromatic hydrocarbons | | + | |
| Radiation * | | + | |
| Radium | | + | |
| Radon | | + | |
| Silica | + | + | + |
| Silicone | + | | + |
| Sulfur dioxide * | ? | + | |
| Toluene 2,4-diisocyanate | + | | |
| Toxic oil (? aniline derivative) * | | | + |
| Trichloroethylene | | + | |
| Vinyl chloride | + | | + |
| Zinc | fumes | + | |
| Various medications * | + | + | + |

Source: ATSDR Toxicological Profiles, HAZDAT database.
* ATSDR Toxicological Profiles not yet available.

substances health effects database HAZDAT (HAZDAT 1993). A review of health effects data associated with substances found at hazardous waste sites concluded that immune effects were likely adverse health outcomes from direct contact with chemical substances, and that the immune system was one of the five organ systems most sensitive to chronic, low-dose exposure to chemical toxicants[8]. Table 2 lists substances associated with immune effects in humans or animals, obtained by reviewing ATSDR Toxicological Profiles prepared for hazardous substances commonly found at facilities on the CERCLA

National Priorities List. Several toxicants with documented immune effects are listed but do not yet have ATSDR Toxicologic Profiles.

## IMMUNE TEST BATTERY

Immune tests proposed for the first tier or basic immune test panel by the three workgroups of the ATSDR Immune Test Battery Workshop. The first tier of tests comprises a basic screening panel to be included in a general assessment of toxic effects on the immune system in a population study (Table 3).

**Table 3.** Immune tests proposed for basic panel by the three workgroups of the ATSDR Immune Test Battery Workshop (1992). A complete blood count (CBC) with a 5-part differential is performed on all participants.

| Test | Age Group | Reference Range |
|---|---|---|
| Total lymphocyte count | 1 - 6 years<br>7 - 14 years<br>8 - 21 years<br>> 21 years | 1,800 - 9,800 cells/mm$^3$<br>2,000 - 6,000 cells/mm$^3$<br>1,350 - 4,500 cells/mm$^3$<br>1,500 - 4,000 cells/mm$^3$ |
| Immunoglobulins G, A, M | See Table 8 | Results from ATSDR multisite studies |
| CD4/CD8 Ratio | All ages | >0.7 (only low values are currently clinically interpretable) |
| CD4 | All ages | >400 cells/mm$^3$ |
| Rheumatoid factor | All ages | Waaler titer <1:40 |
| C Reactive protein | All ages | < 1.0 mg/dL |
| Antinuclear antibody | All ages (> prevalence in older persons) | Negative at ≤ 1:80 |
| Antithyroglobulin antibody | All ages | Method dependent, age dependent, normally <1:10. |

## ADULT ENVIRONMENTAL NEUROBEHAVIORAL TEST BATTERY

In September 1991, ATSDR convened a workshop to advise on the selection of neurobehavioral tests for inclusion in a neurobehavioral test battery. After reviewing the results of the 1991 workshop and various other information sources, ATSDR selected thirteen tests for their Adult Environmental Neurobehavioral Test Battery (AENTB) (Table 4) to identify neurotoxic disorders[9].

ATSDR uses the AENTB to evaluate population groups (not individuals) for adverse nervous system effects produced by exposures to hazardous waste sites. The tests were selected to be used in field study conditions with relatively portable equipment and for administration by persons without specialized training in neurobehavioral testing. Experience has shown that the AENTB can be administered, on average, in 45-55 minutes, and that it is well tolerated by study participants. It should be emphasized that the AENTB is for population screening, and is not appropriate for use in diagnosing

**Table 4**. ATSDR Adult environmental neurobehavioral test battery and average time needed for administration

| Neurobehavioral Test | Average time required (minutes) |
|---|---|
| Acuity and Contrast Sensitivity Tests [two tests/one device] | 4.1 |
| Farnsworth D-15 Color Vision Test (Desaturated) | 5.6 |
| Vibrotactile Threshold | 4.4 |
| Santa Ana | 6.7 |
| Dynamometer | 2.3 |
| Raven Progressive Matrices | 6.8 |
| Symbol Digit | 7.0 |
| NES Tapping Test (one hand) | 2.2 |
| Simple Reaction Time | 10.7 |
| Serial Digit Learning | 3.5 |
| Symbol Digit Delayed Recall Test | included above |
| Vocabulary | 3.2 |
| NES Mood Scale | 2.8 |

specific individual complaints. The AENTB was first used by ATSDR during the summer of 1993, and results from this study are not yet available. Extensive training of study investigators and AENTB administrators is required prior to beginning the study. ATSDR has also employed a scientist with extensive experience in neurobehavioral testing to oversee the training and to audit the test administrators during the study.

If a population exposed to excessive levels of pesticides were to be investigated, a field study would certainly employ a similar, but unexposed, comparison population and both groups would receive a questionnaire addressing current and past health problems (symptom and disease prevalence questionnaire), specific questions designed to address the confounders for the tests included in both the AENTB and tier 1 immune test battery, and for any other biomarker test battery used. If indicated, serum levels of specific pesticides, as well as serial acetylcholinesterase levels would be used in conjunction with the biomarker test batteries. A questionnaire addressing household and occupational use of pesticides would also be administered.

## MAGNITUDE OF THE POPULATION'S EXPOSURE TO PESTICIDES

Definitive data on the extent and severity of the pesticide exposure is not readily available due to underreporting, failure to recognize pesticide related health problems on the part of the public and by physicians, and by the difficulty in determining if a specific effect is truly the result of exposure to pesticides. In occupational exposure there is often reluctance on the part of employer or employee to report a problem. The frequency with which pesticide exposure occurs to individuals or small groups can only be roughly estimated from studying the number of calls made to regional poison control centers or to a national pesticide incident referral center such as the National Pesticide

**Table 5.** Calls received and reported health effects: 1984 to October 1, 1993 by the National Pesticide Telecommunication Network

| Year | Total calls | Serious calls | Chemical sensitivity | Peripheral neuropathy | Death |
|---|---|---|---|---|---|
| 1984 | 9,723 | 2,393 | 67 | 105 for 1984-90 | 687 for 1984-90 (84 humans) |
| 1985 | 14,827 | 2504 | 43 | | |
| 1986 | 18,327 | 3,004 | 87 | | |
| 1987 | 25,780 | 4,516 | 67 | | |
| 1988 | 24,555 | 4,227 | 75 | | |
| 1989 | 33,825 | 4,429 | 94 | | |
| 1990 | 53,598* | 4,305 | 75 | | |
| 1991 | 33,239 | 3,556 | 101 | 12 | 106 (13 human) |
| 1992 | 37,394 | 3,710 | 58 | 6 | 94 (10 human) |
| 1993 (9 mo) | 22,098 | 1,649 | 38 | 3 | 58 (4 human) |

* Mercury paint scare inflated the number of calls

Telecommunication Network (Table 5). This data suffers from reporting bias and inability to classify the conditions due to the limitations of a telephone interview.

## OTHER ATSDR BIOMARKER TEST BATTERIES

The other ATSDR screening biomarker test batteries will not be discussed, but are listed for the sake of completeness. The second and third tier test batteries are also provided. These are used to further define the health problems in a population that was found to have significant abnormalities on initial biomarker screening.

### Tier 1: Hepatobiliary System Basic Screening Test Panel

Aspartate aminotransferase (AST or SGOT)
Alanine aminotransferase (ALT or SPGT)
Gammaglutamyl transferase (GGT)
Alkaline phosphatase (AP)
Fasting bile acids
Triglycerides
Cholesterol
Glucose

### Tier 1: Renal System Basic Screening Panel

Serum creatinine
Serum blood urea nitrogen (BUN)
Serum electrolytes (sodium, potassium, chloride, bicarbonate)

Urinalysis (routine dipstick with microscopic examination)
Urine osmolarity (early morning collection)
N-acetylglucosamine (NAGA)
Beta-2-microglobulin

**Tier 2: Renal System Tests for Specialized Studies**

Glomerular filtration rate (GFR)
24-hour total protein
Creatinine clearance
Kidney stone profile

Glomerular filtration rate (GFR) is the most sensitive of the documented tests for renal function. By using current procedures for GFR determinations, the test can also assess perfusion and tubular uptake. Study subjects with abnormal results on these tests should be referred for individual medical evaluation.

**Tier 3: Renal System Tests for Research Applications**

Kidney biopsy

**Tier 2: Immune System Tests for Specialized Studies**

**Humoral Dysfunction**
Serum immunoglobulin M (IgM)
Serum immunoglobulin A (IgA)
Serum protein electrophoresis
Bone marrow biopsy and examination

**Hypersensitivity Reactions**
Serum total immunoglobulin E (IgE)
Serum antigen-specific IgE ("RAST")
Skin tests for immediate hypersensitivity

## PRIORITY HEALTH CONDITIONS: AREAS OF APPLIED RESEARCH

The areas of applied research selected by ATSDR are:

1. Evaluations of the occurrence of adverse health effects in specific populations. This will include the evaluation of the incidence or prevalence of a disease, disease symptoms, self-reported health concerns, or biological markers of disease, susceptibility, or exposure; and ecologic epidemiology studies.

2. Identification of risk factors for adverse health effects, relevant to NPL sites, in populations. This will include hypothesis generated cohort or case-control studies on potentially affected populations to identify (1) any links between exposure and adverse health effects and (2) those risk factors which may be affected by prevention actions.

3. Development of methods for the diagnosis of adverse health effects in populations. This will include medical research for the identification and validation of new biological tests to evaluate disease occurrence in potentially impacted populations.

4. Diagnosis of adverse health effects in individuals. This will include clinical based research to identify and evaluate diagnostic and treatment regimens which may benefit persons developing adverse health effects resulting from exposure to hazardous substances.

## FUTURE DIRECTIONS

The recent association of pesticide residues in human serum with breast cancer is an example of the potential for previously unsuspected adverse health effects due to pesticides. This association, if upheld, may also signal that studies of other health outcomes and their relation to pesticide exposure may be studied in population groups in the future. Biomarker test batteries require validation against long term health outcome studies in the populations tested. Reference ranges, standardized test methodology, and study of normal variation in test results have become available recently for many of the tests that are now included in the test batteries. As this information is developed on some of the newer tests, they may be used in the screening test battery as a replacement for a less sensitive or specific test, or added as an additional test. Tests now in the screening test batteries may be deleted if there is difficulty with methodology or if poor predictive value for the test is found.

Only after more experience is gained with the administration of test batteries, with the analysis of results, and ultimately with the determination of the predictive value of the test batteries, will the role of biomarker screening of populations for adverse health effects be better understood.

## REFERENCES


1. Wogan, G.N. *et al.*, Biochemical and cellular markers of chemical exposure and preclinical indicators of disease, *in:* "Human health and the environment some research needs - report of the Third Task Force for Research Planning in Environmental Health Sciences", DHHS publication No. (NIH) 86-1277. pp 203-267 (1984).
2. Committee on Biologic Markers of the National Research Council Biologic Markers in Environmental Health Research, *Environ. Health Perspect.* 74:3-9 (1987).
3. U.S. Department of Health and Human Services, Public Health Service, Agency for Toxic Substances and Disease Registry, Study of symptom and disease prevalence, Caldwell Systems, Inc. hazardous waste incinerator, Caldwell county, North Carolina, ATSDR, Atlanta, NTIS PB93-231041 (1993).
4. U.S. Department of Health and Human Services, Public Health Service, Agency for Toxic Substances and Disease Registry, Priority Health Conditions, ATSDR, Atlanta (1993).
5. Pepys, J., Allergens and allergy: Factors involved in allergy to low molecular weight chemicals, *Adv. Biosci.* 74:271-79 (1989).
6. ATSDR, Notice of the revised priority list of hazardous substances for toxicological profiles, *Fed. Regist.* October 17, 1991; 56:52166 (1991).
7. Buffler, P.A., Crane, M., and Key, M.M., Possibilities of detecting health effects by studies of populations exposed to chemicals from waste disposal sites, *Environ. Health Perspect.* 62:423-456 (1985).
8. Hutchinson, L.J., Amler, R.W., Lybarger, J.A. and Chappell, W., Neurobehavioral test batteries for use in environmental health field studies, U.S. Department of Health and Human Services, Public Health Service, ATSDR, Atlanta (1992).

# APPENDICES

# REVISED GUIDANCE DOCUMENT FOR THE CONDUCT OF FIELD STUDIES OF EXPOSURE TO PESTICIDES IN USE

Graham Chester

ZENECA Agrochemicals
Stewardship and Safety Department
Fernhurst, Haslemere
Surrey, U.K. GU27 3JE

## INTRODUCTION

The evaluation of worker exposure to pesticides is an integral part of risk assessment, both for product safety and regulatory assessment purposes and for post-registration surveillance of pesticides in use. The purpose of this document is to review and compare the available methods for measuring pesticide exposure and to provide guidance on the design of studies for the determination of exposure to, and absorption of, pesticides by workers involved in their use.

The document is not intended to cover biological effect monitoring, which may be used as an adjunct to exposure or absorbed dose measurement. Non-occupational exposure to pesticides and the exposure of pesticide manufacturing and formulation workers are also beyond the scope of this document and will not be addressed.

Annexes provide details on methods for the evaluation of exposure and absorbed dose and on quality control and quality assurance. A glossary of important terms is also appended.

## RATIONALE FOR GUIDELINES ON THE CONDUCT OF WORKER EXPOSURE STUDIES

The essential components of a quantitative risk assessment for workers involved in pesticide use are a detailed evaluation of the toxicity of the pesticide, an estimate or measurement of the exposure and/or amount of pesticide absorbed by the workers as a consequence of its use and the likelihood of the expression of any toxicological effect in the workers. Although the evaluation of the toxicity of new pesticides is conducted according to internationally accepted guidelines using harmonized methods and protocols, no such internationally accepted guidelines exist for measuring exposure (although there are different nationally agreed approaches). This guidance document therefore proposes harmonized methods and approaches for the quantitative evaluation of exposure.

*Methods of Pesticide Exposure Assessment*, Edited by
P.B. Curry *et al.*, Plenum Press, New York, 1995

Guidelines and standard protocols for the measurement of exposure have been published previously; notable examples are the World Health Organization (WHO) standard protocol (WHO, 1982) and the U.S. Environmental Protection Agency (EPA) guidelines on applicator/operator exposure (U.S. EPA, 1987). Since their publication, there has been a marked shift in emphasis in regulatory risk assessment in several countries to take account of the extent of occupational exposure and, in particular, the absorbed dose of the compound in question. This shift has led to the development of more sophisticated approaches and methods, notably the increasing use of biological monitoring to measure the extent of absorption of pesticides, interpreted with the aid of pharmacokinetics data from human volunteer studies. The increased use of biological monitoring has developed from the traditional use of biological effect monitoring to assess health effects or modification of normal biochemical indices in workers. There is therefore a need to draw together and review the available methods and present a standardized approach.

## THE TIER APPROACH

A tier approach to risk assessment for pesticides has been discussed by experts at international workshops in The Netherlands and Canada (Henderson et al., 1993; Carmichael, 1995). Emphasis is placed on maximum flexibility to enable the investigator to choose the most appropriate means of estimating or measuring the exposure to, or absorbed dose of, a pesticide.

Within the tier approach, generic exposure data from published databases are compared with no-observed-effect levels from subchronic oral dosing toxicity studies or subacute dermal toxicity studies to see whether the predicted exposure leads to an acceptable margin of safety, in which case there is no need for further investigation (Tier 1). Several databases have been developed, such as the North American Pesticide Handlers Exposure Database (PHED, 1992), the U.K. Predictive Operator Exposure Model (Martin, 1990), the German model (Lundehn et al., 1992) and the Dutch model (van Hemmen, 1992). In the European Community, a database and model that will take European agriculture into consideration are under development (Watts and Chen, 1995).

If dermal absorption data are available, they can be used to refine the estimate of absorbed dose (Tier 2). Exposure mitigation measures (e.g. protective clothing) can also be taken into account. If margins of safety are inadequate based on generic exposure and dermal absorption data, then a study to measure exposure and/or absorbed dose must be done (Tier 3).

A field study must also be considered for use patterns for which no acceptable generic exposure data are available, if it is judged that generating additional exposure data alone will improve the quality of the risk assessment. It may instead be prudent to consider a biological monitoring approach, as absorbed dose data, if interpreted with the aid of experimental human pharmacokinetics data, are likely to be more accurate than the estimate of absorption given by exposure data and correction for dermal absorption. If the risk assessment still indicates excessive exposure, further risk mitigation factors may be considered to reduce the absorbed dose to an acceptable level.

## REVIEW AND COMPARISON OF METHODOLOGY

### Previous Reviews

Early extensive reviews of methodology were published by Durham and Wolfe (1962), Wolfe (1976) and Davis (1980). These reviews, particularly the methodology of Durham and Wolfe (1962), formed the basis of the WHO standard protocol for the measurement of exposure (WHO, 1975, 1982). The first WHO protocol (1975) was aimed primarily at the measurement of exposure to, and absorption of, organophosphorus insecticides and included the Durham and Wolfe (1962) "patch" methodology to estimate dermal exposure. The revised WHO protocol (1982) was designed to assess all classes of pesticides and included an alternative method for the measurement of dermal exposure (the "whole body" clothing technique) as well as an overview of biological monitoring as a means of measuring absorption arising from all routes of exposure. This revised protocol formed the basis of the U.S. National Agricultural Chemicals Association (NACA) guidelines for mixer-loader-applicator exposure studies (Mull and McCarthy, 1986), although the NACA guidelines placed primary emphasis on the use of the Durham and Wolfe (1962) "patch" methodology, with scant reference to the more recently developed "whole body" technique that had figured prominently in the revised WHO protocol.

In 1985, NACA also published guidelines for the conduct of field biological monitoring studies as a means of measuring the absorption of pesticides (NACA, 1985). Both the EPA (U.S. EPA, 1987) and NACA guidelines contained detailed and useful reviews of the advantages and limitations of the various approaches to the measurement of exposure to, and absorption of, pesticides. More recently, the International Group of National Associations of Manufacturers of Agrochemical Products (GIFAP) published a position paper on broad aspects of monitoring studies in the assessment of worker exposure to pesticides (GIFAP, 1990). These guidelines were intended to inform the non-specialist of the various approaches to exposure/absorption evaluation and their significance. They were not intended to give detailed descriptions of the various monitoring techniques or to recommend a specific approach.

Curry and Iyengar (1992) reviewed and compared the currently available guidelines (published and unpublished) for the evaluation of exposure of individuals using pesticides or exposed to pesticide residues in indoor and outdoor environments. Harmonized exposure and biological monitoring guidelines (and the tier approach to evaluation) were proposed in a workshop involving international experts held in The Netherlands (Chester, 1993; Henderson et al., 1993). The Worker Health and Safety Branch of the California Environmental Protection Agency published a guidance document on the preparation of pesticide exposure assessment documents (Thongsinthusak et al., 1993). The document gives information on default values for an exposure assessment, such as body surface areas, body weights, ventilation rates and clothing protection factors, and describes facets of the risk assessment process in California in detail.

Fenske (1993) evaluated the relevance of current dermal exposure sampling methods within the context of a dermal exposure assessment strategy for hazardous chemical substances in general.

## Overview of Methods for Measuring Dermal Exposure (see Annex I for details)

**Patch Method.** In the patch method, the potential contamination of the workers' skin and clothing is measured using a variable number of absorbent cloth or paper patches attached to defined areas of the body, inside and outside clothing. The patches are the so-called "dosimeters" in "passive dosimetry" and act as a collection medium for the pesticide. After a defined or measured period of exposure, the patches are removed and analyzed for pesticide content. In many published studies, the number of patches used per worker represented about 8% of the total body area of approximately 2 $m^2$. The quantity of a pesticide on a patch of known area is related to the area of limb or other body part using standard body part surface areas (U.S. EPA, 1987; see also Table A-1 in Annex I), assuming that the pesticide has been uniformly deposited over the body part. This assumption is perhaps the principal disadvantage of the patch technique, as the extrapolation of the value given by the limit of quantification (LOQ) to the total body part may give a substantial under- or overestimate of exposure. This disadvantage can be addressed in part by increasing the number of patches located on body parts predicted to receive significant exposure. Individual body part exposure values are then added to give a total potential dermal exposure, expressed in mg/h, mg/d or mg/kg product handled or applied.

In the WHO protocol, fewer patches are recommended (representing only 3%, instead of 8%, of the body area), as only the pesticide contacting the normally unclothed area of skin — e.g. head, neck, hands, forearm — is used to calculate actual exposure. In temperate climates, however, about 10% of the total body area is normally unprotected during use of pesticides and other agricultural activities. Furthermore, normal work clothing, such as cotton trousers or shirts, is absorbent and may retain and allow penetration of a proportion of the pesticide. Therefore, it is necessary to estimate exposure to the covered areas of the body as well as exposure to the unclothed areas.

To do this, the amount of pesticide penetration is often measured using patches attached beneath the clothing. Without such inside patches, an estimate of penetration of normal clothing is usually proposed. However, penetration of clothing by pesticides is a highly variable process that is influenced by such factors as the type of formulation (liquid or solid), the amount or volume of deposition on the clothing, the dampness of the clothing, the location of deposition (e.g. seams) and the type of fabric. Further uncertainties are introduced by the method of sampling.

The patch method may give significant under- or overestimates of exposure, depending on whether the patches have captured the non-uniform, random deposition of concentrate splashes or spray droplets. This limitation applies equally to crop reentry procedures, such as harvesting, where contact with the crop is not a uniform process. One solution to the problem of non-uniform exposure is an increase in sample size. The development of the Pesticide Handlers Exposure Database (PHED, 1992) is an attempt to give more accurate estimates of exposures to different body regions. Despite its readily apparent limitations, the patch method can serve as a cost-effective method for evaluating pesticide exposure, particularly in comparative studies.

**Whole Body Method.** One means of overcoming the inherent problems of the patch method is the use of lightweight coveralls or similar type of clothing in the whole body method (WHO, 1982; Abbott et al., 1987). This method is more convenient in a practical sense, in that investigators do not need to attach patches to the clothing and skin of workers, which is a time-consuming process. Exposure of the head is assessed by incorporating a hood into the coverall or using a separate cotton hat. Any additional protective clothing and equipment recommended for the product under study are worn over the sampling clothing, thus enabling an evaluation of their protection. Cotton undergarments (long pants and long-sleeved T-shirts) may also be worn beneath the normal work clothing to estimate dermal exposure of the entire covered part of the body. The use of the whole body method overcomes the problem posed by the assumption of uniformity of deposition in the patch method, as most of the pesticide is likely to be captured if woven protective materials are used as the sampling medium. Furthermore, it is not necessary to extrapolate from small target areas to larger body regions. For these reasons, the whole body method is believed to give a more accurate estimate of potential dermal exposure, although this has not yet been verified.

A variant of the whole body method is the use of clothing that represents what the workers would normally wear under the prevailing conditions as dermal dosimeters (Chester et al., 1990). This method is particularly applicable to field studies involving concurrent evaluation of dermal exposure and absorbed dose with biological monitoring. Whereas the patch and standard whole body methods place sampling media between the pesticide and the clothing or skin (thus acting as a barrier interfering with the normal process of skin contamination and percutaneous absorption), the advantage of this method is that the capture, retention and penetration properties of the normal work clothing are mimicked as closely as possible. It is important, therefore, to have a good appreciation of the range of normal work clothing worn by the worker population under study. The selection of sampling clothing should err on the cautious side by utilizing the minimum clothing that might be worn under the prevailing conditions. Therefore, the assessment of residual clothing contamination and transfer to the skin beneath the clothing is as realistic as possible. This method is particularly relevant for northern European and North American temperate countries, where the typical work clothing consists of a T-shirt, long-sleeved shirt, socks and long trousers and/or coveralls. Such clothing may also be relevant for some tropical countries.

The variant of the whole body method can be used to estimate dermal exposure concurrently with the use of biological monitoring to measure absorbed dose, as it does not interfere with the normal process of contamination and percutaneous absorption. Actual exposure of the skin beneath the clothing can be estimated by taking account of the ratio of outer to inner clothing penetration or transfer of the pesticide. An obvious limitation is that it has to be assumed that the permeation and transfer properties of the outer and inner clothing are the same. For analytical considerations, it may be necessary to use non-coloured, white materials such as cotton or cotton/polyester mixtures. As in the standard whole body method, the clothing is sectioned into individual body parts and analyzed separately to determine the regional distribution of total potential and actual dermal exposure.

It should be noted that little attempt has been made to validate methods for the monitoring of dermal exposure (e.g. using biological monitoring to compare the derivations of absorbed dose). Until the methods are validated, they should all be regarded as providing only an indicative measure of dermal exposure. The challenge is to find a sampling medium that mimics skin in its pesticide capture and retention characteristics and thus can predict actual exposure. Given that biological monitoring for determination of absorbed dose does not lend itself to all pesticides — e.g. because of extensive metabolism or routes of elimination other than the kidney — there remains a strong need to develop and refine exposure methods.

**Use of Fluorescent Tracers and Visible Dyes to Quantify Exposure by Analysis or Video Imaging.**[1] Dermal exposure can be quantified directly by measuring the deposition of fluorescent materials or visible dyes on the clothing and/or skin. The fluorescent tracer or dye can be substituted and extracted from passive dosimeters and analyzed in the same way as the pesticide. By adjusting for concentration differences, an estimate of exposure to the pesticide can be obtained.

A recent technical advance is the development of a fluorescent tracer/video imaging technique (Fenske et al., 1986 a,b; Fenske, 1990), which involves the incorporation of a fluorescent tracer in a pesticide formulation and subsequent visual and quantitative analysis using a video imaging technique. This method reveals non-uniform patterns of exposure that escape detection by the patch technique. It has also demonstrated that exposure can occur beneath protective clothing. An important advantage of this technique is that the skin serves as a collection medium, rather than dosimeter patches or clothing. The main limitations of this method are the assumptions that the relative transfer of the tracer and the pesticide in the field and their permeation of the clothing are equivalent. However, these assumptions are analogous to those involving generic exposure data: that is, the exposure to a pesticide measured under a given set of conditions is assumed to represent that associated with a second pesticide

[1] This method is not discussed further in Annex I.

under the same conditions. Possible differences in the relative transfer of the tracer and the pesticide can be assessed by conducting ancillary studies. The technique is particularly useful for the training of operators by demonstrating the extent of their contamination, thus allowing them to modify their working practices to reduce exposure. A second-generation imaging system with improved exposure quantification is now available (Fenske et al., 1990).

If an investigator chooses to use a tracer compound or visible dye, he/she should validate its performance and suitability as a surrogate for the intended measurement before the field study. Apart from the usual criteria of quality control (QC) acceptability that are applicable to all pesticides, the surrogate compound should not significantly alter the physical properties of the formulation or spray mixture. The key question regarding the utility of a tracer or dye is whether it impacts, is retained by or penetrates clothing alongside the pesticide of interest. Clearly, it can be used only in ambient exposure monitoring and not in biological monitoring (although it can be used with concurrent biological monitoring of a pesticide). Its greatest utility is probably as a substitute in exposure studies for pesticides that are unstable during the sampling and analytical phases.

The main advantages and limitations of the above methods for estimating dermal exposure (other than hand exposure) are summarized in Table 1.

**Table 1.** Main advantages and limitations of the methods for estimating dermal exposure [1]

| Dermal exposure method | Main advantages | Main limitations | Use with concurrent biological monitoring |
|---|---|---|---|
| Patch | Ease of analysis | Assumes uniform deposition | Yes |
| Whole body | No body region size or surface area correction necessary | Cumbersome analysis | No |
| Variant of whole body | Collects most pesticide not reaching skin | Cumbersome analysis | Yes |
| Dyes/video imaging | 1. Visual and quantitative analysis (conventionally or video imaging)<br>2. Measures exposure directly from skin (video imaging) | Assumes equivalent clothing permeation by dye and pesticide | Yes |

[1] Methods for estimating dermal exposure of the hands are summarized in Table 2.

**Hand Exposure.** Monitoring of hand exposure may be the most important measurement in a dermal exposure study. The contribution of the hands to total exposure has been well documented by many investigators, using a variety of methods (U.S. EPA, 1987). The methods include the use of lightweight absorbent gloves or sections cut from gloves, swabbing or rinsing the hands in various solvents (U.S. EPA, 1987) and using the normal process of washing the hands with soap and water to provide an estimate of exposure during concurrent biological monitoring (Chester et al., 1990). All these approaches have their advantages and limitations, and it is not possible to evaluate the accuracy of any procedure. The best that can be achieved for a hand wash or hand rinse method is a laboratory validation of the efficiency of recovery of material from the hands of human volunteers. This has been investigated recently by Fenske and Lu (1994) for the insecticide chlorpyrifos using a solvent hand rinse method. Their findings suggest that exposure to pesticides that are well absorbed by, or adsorbed to, the skin cannot be estimated accurately by a hand rinse method.

The U.S. EPA (1987) stated that the use of gloves as a monitoring technique may result in a significant overestimation of total dermal exposure, owing to their capacity to retain more of the pesticide than would be retained by the skin. Gloves also contain foreign materials, which, unless pre-extracted, may be co-extracted with the pesticide. This may be a problem at low levels of contamination, although the levels of glove contamination due to dirt and grease are a greater problem in this respect. The hands also tend to incur significant levels of pesticide contamination, and low-level interference may not be as significant a problem as inferred by the U.S. EPA (1987).

Washing the hands with a solvent is considered by some to disrupt skin barrier function and enhance percutaneous absorption of the pesticide. The U.S. EPA (1987) claimed that there is little actual evidence for this and recommended washing using the bag rinse method developed by Durham and Wolfe (1962). The EPA's preference for the bag rinse technique over washing of the hands in a bowl appears to be because the bag rinse method is a standardized procedure and because the data generated by it are consistent with those in the existing database.

In conclusion, it is not possible to recommend one method for estimating hand exposure over another insofar as accuracy of measurement is concerned.

Where exposure measurements and biological monitoring are to be conducted concurrently, a hand-washing procedure involving soap and water is proposed for use whenever the workers would normally wash their hands and where it is feasible to do so. The rationale for this proposal is that when absorption is assessed, there should be no interference with the normal process of dermal contamination and percutaneous absorption. Therefore, the use of absorbent gloves or a solvent washing or rinsing technique is inappropriate, as the gloves would retain pesticide otherwise available for absorption and the solvents could potentially disrupt the barrier function of the skin. By performing a hand wash with ordinary soap and water whenever the worker chooses to wash his/her hands, this normal process of contamination and absorption is not unduly influenced, and the investigator is simply collecting what would be disposed of under normal circumstances. This technique may provide an estimate of hand exposure, particularly if the worker chooses to wash at frequent intervals, such as after mixing or at meal breaks. The efficiency of the washing procedure for removal of the pesticide can be gauged by laboratory validation studies using the chosen soap and the normal process of hand washing. The major disadvantage is the loss of standardization between workers owing to the variable number of hand washes. Any protective gloves worn, together with any protective glove washings, may also be taken for analysis to determine the potential exposure of the hands. An important analytical consideration is the laboratory validation of the extraction efficiency of the chosen soap and water prior to the field study. It is recommended that the soap be standardized for all workers in the study to ensure consistency of extraction efficiency.

The main advantages and limitations of the methods for estimating the dermal exposure of the hands are summarized in Table 2.

**Methods for Measuring Inhalation Exposure (see Annex I for details)**

One of the earliest but most complete reviews of the methodology for field monitoring of airborne pesticides was by Lewis (1976). Van Dyk and Visweswariah (1975) had previously reviewed the media available for collection of pesticides, but with particular emphasis on static environmental sampling. A personal air sampling technique is the method of choice for the determination of airborne concentrations of pesticides in

**Table 2.** Main advantages and limitations for estimating the dermal exposure of the hands

| Hand exposure method | Main advantages | Main limitations | Use with concurrent biological monitoring |
|---|---|---|---|
| Absorbent gloves | Ease of use | Possible overestimation of exposure | No |
| Solvent/swab rinse wash | Standardized method enabling comparison with most previous data | 1. May disrupt barrier function of skin<br>2. Possible underestimation of exposure | No |
| Hand wash (soap and water) | Does not interfere with process of skin contamination and absorption | 1. Loss of standardization between workers<br>2. Possible underestimation of exposure | Yes |

the breathing zones of workers. Several techniques are available, ranging from the use of gauze pads in respirators, pioneered by Durham and Wolfe (1962), to the use of solid adsorbents and filter cassettes attached to battery-powered personal sampling pumps. A personal sampling technique involving sampling devices mounted in the breathing zone and sampling pumps is preferred. Use of the personal air sampler permits any label-recommended use of respirators or dust masks, but it does not measure inhalation exposure of workers wearing respiratory protection.

The choice of sampling medium is dictated by the nature of the pesticide, in that a suitable filter cassette or sampling head should be used for spray particulates and a solid adsorbent material for volatile compounds. An example of a suitable personal sampling head is the Institute of Occupational Medicine's (IOM) personal sampling head, designed specifically to collect the inspirable fraction (all material capable of being drawn into the nose and mouth), which is the most relevant fraction to measure (Vincent and Mark, 1987). To use this device, a sampling flow rate of 2 L/min is necessary. Examples of suitable adsorbent materials for some volatile compounds are activated charcoal, "Tenax" and XAD-2 resins mounted in stainless steel or glass tubes. The choice of material should be determined by analytical retention (trapping efficiency) and extractability studies before monitoring.

It may be necessary to sample concurrently for particulates and vapour, in which case the filter sampling head is mounted in front of the vapour trap in a "sampling train." This train allows retention on the resin of any vapour stripped off the filter. The material on the filter can be analyzed gravimetrically and/or chemically, and an estimate can be made of the pesticide content of the particulate sample. Where use of such a sampling train is indicated, laboratory validation of the sampling efficiency, particularly of the adsorbent resin, is necessary, owing to the possibility that material may be stripped from the resin by the relatively high flow rate (typically 1-4 L/min).

The measurement of the inspirable fraction and the use of adsorbent resins for the vapour component are recommended as the method of choice for estimating exposure by inhalation. The advantages and limitations of this method are summarized in Table 3.

**Methods for Measuring the Absorbed Dose (Biological Monitoring) (see Annex I for details)**

Biological monitoring is a method of evaluating the absorption of chemicals by

**Table 3.** Main advantages and limitations of the method for estimating exposure by inhalation

| Inhalation exposure method | Main advantage | Main limitation | Use with concurrent biological monitoring |
|---|---|---|---|
| Personal air sampler (inspirable/ vapour) | Measures potential inhalation and subsequent oral ingestion | Need to estimate ventilation rate | Yes |

measuring the chemical or its metabolites in body fluids, usually urine, blood or exhaled breath. Biological effect monitoring (use of biomarkers) has been used in the chemical industry for many years to assess health effects or modification of normal biochemical indices in workers as a consequence of exposure. In the context of pesticides, it has been used most frequently for assessing exposure to organophosphorus compounds by measuring blood cholinesterase activity (see, for example, Peoples and Knaak, 1982).

Analysis of body fluids and excreta, most commonly blood and urine, for the parent compound or its metabolites can provide both a qualitative and a quantitative measurement of absorbed dose for those pesticides considered suitable candidates for biological monitoring. This measurement of absorbed dose is perceived as the principal advantage of biological monitoring over ambient exposure monitoring, as it evaluates actual, rather than potential, absorption. It integrates absorption from all possible routes of exposure: dermal, inhalation and primary and secondary oral ingestion. However, differentiating the contributions to the absorbed dose from different aspects of the work can be done only with a specifically tailored study design. For details and wider-ranging discussions of biological monitoring, the reader is referred to Van Heemstra-Lequin and Van Sittert (1986), Wang et al. (1989) and Henderson et al. (1993).

In order to obtain quantitative data on the amount of pesticide absorbed by workers, it is necessary to understand the metabolism and pharmacokinetics of the compound in humans. This requirement has been dealt with in detail by Woollen (1993). Field biological monitoring studies that have utilized or described human metabolism and pharmacokinetics data, either to interpret the absorbed dose or used as an adjunct, include those on the herbicide fluazifop-butyl (Chester and Hart, 1986) and 2,4-D amine (Grover et al., 1986; Ritter and Franklin, 1989). Data from such human volunteer dosing studies enable a correct field sampling strategy and define the body fluid matrix of choice. Urine is the ideal sampling matrix, as its collection is non-invasive and the collection of 24-hour voids is practicable. It is advisable to check the completeness of 24-hour urine collections by measuring the concentration of creatinine and expressing excretion as g/d. Substantially incomplete collections are readily apparent; they can either be excluded or an allowance made for them — for example, by using a correction factor based upon the average daily urine volume for the individual concerned (Woollen, 1993). Other parameters, such as specific gravity and osmolarity, may also be useful in this respect (Alessio et al., 1985). The utility of creatinine as a tool for checking compliance and in correcting urinary concentrations of excreted substances has been reviewed by Boeniger et al. (1993).

The need for human metabolism and pharmacokinetics data is perceived by some as a major disadvantage of biological monitoring (NACA, 1985). However, this potential disadvantage must be weighed against the more accurate assessment of absorbed dose provided by a properly designed, interpretable biological monitoring study. Such a study may also provide a better understanding of the relevance of the toxicity data to the risk assessment for occupational exposure.

Some pesticides are unstable or highly volatile and therefore are not good candidates for ambient exposure monitoring, despite efforts to accurately assess in-field, storage and transit losses. Biological monitoring should be considered for such pesticides and may, in fact, be the only means of obtaining adequate quantitative data from which the absorbed dose can be derived.

If, for some technical or ethical consideration, a human volunteer study is regarded as impracticable, then the use of animal metabolism and pharmacokinetics data would have to be considered. If metabolism and excretion kinetics for a specific compound are similar in several animal species, then it may be assumed that humans will metabolize and excrete the compound in a similar manner. However, it must be recognized that the assumption carries with it a degree of uncertainty. Clear examples that demonstrate the pitfalls of adopting this approach are described in detail by Woollen (1993). Apart from interspecies differences in metabolism, there is the possibility of dose-dependent differences, pointing to the need for metabolism studies in animals and human volunteers at doses similar to the anticipated workplace exposures. In the absence of human metabolism and pharmacokinetics data, the principal advantage of biological monitoring — i.e. to provide an accurate assessment of the absorbed dose — is reduced.

Certain pesticides may not lend themselves to a biological monitoring strategy — for example, if they are extensively metabolized to a large number of minor metabolites. A minor metabolite does not provide an adequate basis for an accurate assessment of the absorbed dose of the parent compound, particularly if the proportion of the parent compound excreted as the metabolite is subject to interindividual variability. However, depending on the nature of the risk assessment, a minor metabolite can provide some useful information as a "biological indicator" in the absence of more abundant biological monitoring markers.

## QUALITY ASSURANCE/QUALITY CONTROL DATA (see Annex II for details)

Quality assurance/quality control (QA/QC) data on the validity of the analytical methods and on the stability of the pesticide and its metabolites under field, storage and transit conditions are an essential requirement for field studies of occupational exposure.

The process of method development involves the application of chemical principles and laboratory techniques to the reliable analysis of a compound in a specific matrix. It is necessary to demonstrate that reproducible results can be obtained when measuring analytes at the desired level of sensitivity and for all sampling matrices prior to the initiation of field studies.

The process of method validation involves designing and performing experiments to establish the expected accuracy, precision and specificity of a procedure for specific concentration ranges of each analyte of interest in a specific matrix. It includes the determination of a method limit of quantitation (LOQ), the analysis of a range of recovery samples and may include an evaluation of the stability of the analytes in or on the matrices under storage conditions. The necessary LOQ will depend on the toxicological endpoint of interest. At a minimum, the LOQ should be sufficient to assess exposures at the no-observed-effect level divided by an appropriate safety factor. Validation studies should ideally be completed prior to the initiation of a field study.

Laboratory recovery data are generated to determine the efficiency with which the analyte can be recovered from fortified sampling matrices. These data are usually obtained during the method development and method validation processes. Laboratory recoveries reflect losses that may occur during laboratory operations, such as extraction, clean-up and analytical measurement, as well as contamination. It is advisable to include at least one procedural laboratory recovery in each sample analytical run to account for day-to-day variation in the efficiency of the method. Laboratory recoveries are an essential requirement for each study and should cover the range of concentrations anticipated in the field samples.

A storage stability study may also be required and can precede or be conducted concurrently with a field study. Its purpose is to determine the stability of the analytes in or on sampling matrices under the same storage conditions that will be used to store field samples. If at all possible, it is recommended that a storage stability study be conducted prior to the initiation of the field study to determine the maximum duration of storage time that is feasible.

Evaluation of field recovery is essential to enable correction of the test sample data for losses that occur during all phases of sample collection and analysis. Specifically, field recovery samples account for the losses that occur during sample collection, sample handling and storage in the field, transportation from the field to the laboratory, storage in the laboratory, sample extraction and analysis. In addition to field recovery samples, travel recovery samples can be prepared in the field and shipped and stored with the experimental samples. These data provide a basis for estimating the losses that occur during sample shipment and storage as opposed to those that occur during sample collection.

## GENERAL FEATURES OF FIELD STUDY STRATEGY AND DESIGN

The primary aim of a field exposure and/or biological monitoring study is to generate data for use in a risk assessment. This process must also involve characterization of the population at risk and the distribution of exposures within this population (National Academy of Sciences, 1983). The sampling strategy and study design should therefore take account of the need to characterize the central tendency and variability of the exposures incurred by these individuals. There may be extensive prior knowledge of worker populations, working conditions and practices. For products and use patterns for which this is not the case, a useful means of acquiring such information is to conduct a qualitative survey of the working conditions and practices. This helps to identify those worker subgroups and procedures with significant exposure potential. Moreover, it will help determine those sites that should be included in the field study. This information will help in the development of an optimum field study protocol with the best possible study design. This design inevitably must take into account the practical and financial limitations inherent in human studies under arduous and difficult conditions in the field.

Exposure/biological monitoring field studies can be separated into two types: pre- and re-registration studies, and post-registration surveillance studies. Studies of the first type would be conducted in full compliance with the requirements of the anticipated or existing product label — in particular, use of recommended application rates, protective clothing and equipment and procedures for dealing with product spillage. Therefore, the study design would automatically impose certain constraints on the activities of the test subjects, which may, in turn, have some influence on the amount and variability of exposures. Studies of the second type would be done essentially in the interests of good product stewardship and surveillance. Concerns may arise, for example, over some new toxicological findings with a pesticide or because of reported adverse effects on the health of workers, or there may be a need to study the extent of compliance with product label precautions and recommendations. Therefore, the study design would incorporate the need to evaluate exposure under the *actual* conditions of use and would be free of the constraints imposed on pre- or re-registration studies.

Before starting a field study, investigators should consider whether ambient exposure and biological monitoring need to be conducted concurrently. Both may be justified, to provide data for inclusion in generic databases, to examine the relationship between exposure and absorption and to provide a second measurement should one fail. One useful feature of the tier approach (Henderson et al., 1993) is that insight into the likely routes of exposure may be gained from the generic exposure databases, thus enabling a decision on the routes on which to concentrate in the field study. For example, it is well established that mixing, loading and high-volume application of non-volatile pesticides (saturation vapour pressure $<10^{-2}$ Pa; Lundehn et al., 1992), other than wettable powder and dusty granular formulations, do not usually generate significant amounts of inspirable particulates. It therefore seems unnecessary to monitor inhalation exposure in such circumstances.

Other factors that may influence the sampling strategy include possible concern over specific work activities during pesticide use. Passive dosimetry may be more useful than other strategies, in that it enables separate measurements of the respective contributions of these activities to the total exposure. However, if ambient exposure and biological monitoring are conducted concurrently, then these contributions may be assessed simultaneously. Identifying the differences in the magnitude of exposure attributable to these activities permits the use of different regulatory options for mitigating exposure — for example, the recommended use of additional protective equipment during procedures with greater potential for exposure.

The choice of sampling methods for studies in hot and humid climates should be made with due regard to the possible discomfort and encumbrance imposed by passive dosimeters. The use of biological monitoring in these circumstances is advantageous and should be considered provided that the requisite criteria for a scientifically valid study can be met.

If adequate exposure data are available on the pesticide and use pattern in question, biological monitoring may be conducted on the subjects wearing their normal work clothing and any additional protective clothing and equipment required by the label. This approach has the advantage of removing all doubt about possible interference of the exposure sampling dosimeters with the process of skin contamination and absorption.

As stated previously, the emphasis in this document is on maximum flexibility. This applies not only to the different approaches to exposure assessment but also to the specific methodology used to determine the exposure or absorbed dose. For example, the investigator may believe that use of the dermal "patch" method will provide adequate data for his/her purpose. It is essential that a scientifically sound protocol is followed and that the approval of the regulatory authority is sought.

An important consideration is that of the number of measurements of exposure and/or absorbed dose that are needed in the field study. As a general guide, a minimum of 10 subjects is proposed. The choice of number of subjects should be based on a consideration of the likely end use of the data, the nature of any identified toxicological end point, the required level of statistical confidence and the overall manageability of the field study. Where feasible, subjects should be randomly selected from the worker population. It is recommended that a sufficient number of measurements be made in different locations to cover the range of use procedures, conditions and application equipment for which evaluation of exposure and/or absorbed dose is required. These comments also apply to crop reentry procedures; in harvesting, for example, variation in work procedures may be substantial, even within the same crop.

The inherent variability in exposure under field conditions is best addressed by increasing the number of subjects, rather than repeated monitoring of the same individuals; variability between workers is greater than that within the same worker. Equally, consideration should be given to including as many sites as is feasible, rather than repeating measurements on subjects using the same equipment under the same conditions. This applies particularly where location is believed to have a significant impact on the variability of the exposure measurements. Certain types of pesticide application procedure, such as those involving aerial application, render management of the study difficult. In such cases, repeated monitoring of the same individuals is an option, although the limitations of such a choice should be recognized. Should biological monitoring be necessary, a further limitation is introduced, in that interindividual variation in metabolism of the pesticide would be less well evaluated. The duration of the study would be prolonged owing to the possible need to collect urine samples over several days for each individual. As a result, repeat monitoring could not commence until urine collection was complete. These difficulties should be considered if using biological monitoring in such circumstances.

Ideally, the duration of a single measurement of exposure or absorbed dose should be representative of the typical working day, so that there is a greater chance that all the work activities that might result in exposure, such as equipment repair and clean-up, are assessed. This criterion applies particularly to studies involving biological monitoring; unlike ambient exposure data, absorbed dose data may not lend themselves to extrapolation on the basis of time or amount of active ingredient used. In studies involving passive dosimetry and a volatile or unstable pesticide, a shorter monitoring period should be considered, based on a consideration of the physico-chemical properties of the compound. The choice of monitoring duration should take account of the possibility of dosimeter saturation. Ideally, a single set of dosimeters should be used per worker; however, a change of dosimeters during the work day may be necessary if different tasks are to be monitored separately.

The choice of use pattern (including application equipment) should be based on consideration of such factors as whether it is the predominant one for the product or a minor one for which no generic data are available. In pre-registration studies, the product should be used in the study at a representative recommended rate of application and on the likely maximum area of crop treatable in a working day under local conditions. It should also be applied in accordance with all the label recommendations for use. These principles also apply to studies involving crop reentry and for which exposure should be determined after the shortest permissible reentry period (if known). In post-registration surveillance studies, these criteria should not be enforced; this ensures maximum representativity of actual use conditions and exposure variability.

Where the product label recommends the use of protective clothing and/or equipment, such clothing and equipment should be provided to the subjects in pre-registration studies by the supervisory team to ensure standardization. This will aid the scientific interpretation of the data, as the variable of differing standards of protection by different types of protective equipment will have been removed. Including criteria such as these ensures that the exposure and risk assessment for the product are evaluated in accordance with the label recommendations for its regulatory use. However, efforts should be made to ensure that the recommended protective clothing and equipment are practical and realistic to use under local conditions. In post-registration surveillance studies, use of protective clothing and equipment should not be mandatory, although ethical or legal viewpoints on product label recommendations in this respect should be considered.

## TEST SUBJECTS

The test subjects in a field study should be normal workers, rather than inexperienced volunteers. If this is not possible, the use of non-professional personnel may have to be considered, provided that they are given the requisite training in the handling and use of the pesticide and equipment. The limitations of this choice in terms of reducing representativity should be recognized. Males or females may be considered for inclusion in ambient exposure studies. However, in those studies involving biological monitoring, it is preferable that both sexes be included, particularly if it is likely that the product will be used by both sexes, owing to possible sex differences in metabolism and pharmacokinetics.

The informed consent of all subjects should be obtained by providing them with the requisite information on the pesticide in an easily understood form. A consent form should be signed by each subject. Test subjects should not be chosen on the basis of either known careful use of pesticides or good personal hygiene and working practices; they should be representative of the working population under study. Furthermore, they should be told to use the pesticide and carry out work activities according to their normal practice. The subjects should consider themselves to be in normal good health. Consideration should be given to the toxicity of the pesticide and the need for the screening of subjects for any pre-existing conditions that may be affected by use of the pesticide under study. It is useful to give a simple questionnaire to the subjects before a field study to gather information on their experience in the use of pesticides and application equipment, their use of protective equipment and their general health status. It should be made clear to all potential participants that they are free to withdraw from the monitoring study at any time. Consideration should be given to providing the subjects with their individual results.

## MANAGEMENT OF THE STUDY

The field study must be managed and supervised by people trained and experienced in the conduct of exposure studies. Emphasis should be placed upon training and competence of the supervisory team in the field sampling and observational procedures.

## GOOD LABORATORY (FIELD) PRACTICE

The field study should be conducted in accordance with the principles of Good Laboratory Practices (GLP) as applied to field studies and recommended, for example, by the Organisation for Economic Co-operation and Development (OECD, 1992) and others.

# ANNEX I

# PASSIVE DOSIMETRY AND BIOLOGICAL MONITORING METHODS FOR ASSESSMENT OF EXPOSURE AND ABSORBED DOSE

## DERMAL EXPOSURE

### Patch Method

**Patch Description.** The patch dosimeter acts as a barrier to entrap pesticide that would impact on the clothing or, if the patch is located beneath the clothing, would otherwise reach the skin. Therefore, the composition of the patch and its location on each body region should be considered, based on the type of pesticide formulation handled, the application equipment used and the crop.

It is recommended that the collection area of each patch be approximately 10 cm × 10 cm in size.

For liquid pesticide formulations, patches should be made of an appropriate absorbent material such as surgical gauze, paper-making pulp (alpha-cellulose), clothing material, blotter paper or preparative chromatography paper. The patch material should be absorbent enough to retain all liquid residues anticipated to be in contact during an actual field study, as if it were the clothing or the skin, depending on the location of the patches. Multilayer patches can be constructed by stapling together several patches of the same material.

For dry pesticide formulations, patches should be porous enough to collect dusts or dried residues. Surgical gauze is currently the most appropriate collection medium for dry formulations.

The collection medium should be backed by an appropriate impermeable material to prevent the contamination of the patches by residues on the skin or clothing and to prevent seepage through the pad onto the clothing underneath. Suggested backing materials include aluminum foil, polyethylene and glassine paper.

The exposed surface area of the patch should be standardized by placing the patch in a holder envelope with an open window of a standardized area or by trimming the patch to a standard size (i.e. 10 cm × 10 cm) after removing it from the subject.

**Location of Patches.** Inner and outer patches should be attached at the locations listed in Table A-1. These patch placement locations are consistent with the EPA Sub-

**Table A-1.** Surface areas for regions of adult body (80th percentile male) and locations of dermal exposure dosimeters [1]

| Region of body | Surface area ($cm^2$) | Location of dosimeters |
|---|---|---|
| Head and face | 1300 | Head (front of cap, hood) |
| (Face) | (650) | |
| Back of neck | 110 | Back (outside dosimeter) |
| Front of neck (includes "V" of chest) | 150 | Chest (outside dosimeter) |
| Back | 3550 | Back (inside dosimeter) |
| Chest/stomach | 3550 | Chest (inside dosimeter) |
| Upper arms | 2910 | Each upper arm |
| Forearms | 1210 | Each forearm |
| Upper legs | 3820 | Each thigh |
| Lower legs | 2380 | Each lower leg (shin) |
| Feet | 1310 | Each foot or sock |
| Hands | 820 | Absorbent glove or hand wash method used[2] |

Note: Surface areas include both arms, both legs, both hands.

[1] One patch on head, back, chest, each forearm, each upper arm, each thigh and each lower leg.
[2] No surface area calculation is required when either the absorbent glove or the hand wash method is used.

Source: Adapted by U.S. EPA (1987) from Berkow (1931) and U.S. EPA (1985).

division U Guidelines for Applicator Exposure Monitoring (U.S. EPA, 1987). Patch location may vary on a case-by-case basis, however, and additional patches should be placed in areas where, for given conditions, significant exposure is expected. For example, if a worker must carry bags of formulated product, patches may be required on the chest/abdomen area.

A head patch may be used to estimate deposition on the head. The patch may be affixed to the worker's headwear or directly to the head if headwear is not worn.

**Attachment of Patches.** The patches should be securely attached to the skin using suitable material such as surgical tape or sweatbands and/or to the clothing and headwear using safety pins, staples and tape. If attachment to the skin is a concern because of, for example, contact sensitization potential of the tape, consideration should be given to attaching patches to the underside of clothing (inner surface). During attachment, suitable handling methods should be employed to avoid contamination of the patches.

Outside patches should be attached to the outer layer of clothing. Inside patches should not be occluded by the outer patches. They should be placed under the normally worn clothing. They should be attached to the skin or underclothing but not to the clothing used for the attachment of the outer patches.

Every effort should be made to assess areas likely to receive maximum penetration (e.g. seams, openings, etc.) when positioning patches on the specified body areas.

**Patch Removal.** Patches should be replaced immediately if they become saturated or torn; this entails continual observation and frequent examination of the condition of the patches.

If a lengthy time period occurs between monitoring exposures (i.e. morning and evening applications), dosimeters should be replaced between exposures.

Patches should be removed using a suitable method that minimizes the potential for contamination. The patches should be trimmed (if necessary) to a standard size.

### Whole Body Dosimeter Technique

**Dosimeter Description.** The whole body dosimeter acts as a barrier to entrap pesticide that would otherwise contact the clothing or, in the case of an inner dosimeter, would penetrate through the clothing to the skin. The dosimeter should cover all potentially exposed body regions. It should be constructed of suitable absorbent materials, such as cotton or cotton/polyester undergarments, socks, trousers, long-sleeved shirts and coveralls. Garments made of non-absorbent materials may be unsuitable for certain types of formulation. The whole body dosimeter technique may not be suitable for granular or wettable powder pesticide formulations unless the materials are representative of normal clothing in terms of impaction, penetration and retention properties. The materials mentioned above meet this criterion.

The inner whole body dosimeter should be worn under appropriate layers of clothing to represent or mimic the skin. Normal work clothes and other protective equipment should be worn over the dosimeter. This is analogous to the inner patches from the patch technique.

Outer deposition may also be measured to permit comparison of inside and outside contamination and to allow an evaluation of penetration through clothing and protective equipment. The outer dosimeter must not constitute an additional clothing layer over that normally worn and should be handled in a manner similar to that described for the inner whole body dosimeter method.

Exposure to the head, neck and face should be determined by measuring deposition on a cotton hat or cap, on a hood as part of the whole body dosimeter or on a head patch as per the patch technique. Exposure to the face and neck could also be determined through the use of wipe samples.

Exposure to the feet should be estimated from deposition on socks, which are part of the outer deposition dosimeters.

**Donning and Wearing of the Whole Body Dosimeters.** Unused sampling garments, treated in the same manner as in the method validation work (e.g. pre-extracted and laundered), should be issued to the test subjects immediately before the start of the monitoring period. The clothing should be donned in an area free from contamination with the test material or other chemical contaminants and worn throughout the monitoring period, usually the working day or the duration of some specified work activity.

**Removal of Dosimeter.** The dosimeter should be removed and replaced immediately should saturation occur or be anticipated during the work day; this requires continual observation and frequent examination of the condition of the garments. After exposure, the whole body dosimeter should be removed, turned inside out to minimize loss of test material and sectioned for storage, extraction and analysis, using suitable standardized methods that will not result in contamination. If the test material is a granular or powdered product, turning the dosimeter inside out may result in loss through handling; the decision to do this should therefore be considered carefully. This activity should take place in an area free from contamination with the test material and other chemicals. To help minimize cross-contamination after removing the dosimeter from the subject (with assistance from a member of the monitoring team where necessary), individual garment samples should be handled sequentially in terms of contamination potential (i.e. working from low to high contamination). The following outer dosimeter sections are recommended:

Forearms - elbow to wrist
Upper arms - elbow to shoulder
Lower legs - knee to ankle
Upper legs - knee to groin
Chest/torso
Back/torso

These sections can be varied according to the typical clothing worn by the workers and the body parts of interest in terms of distribution of exposure. Inner dosimeters may be analyzed whole, if required. This may minimize the potential inaccuracy of summing individual residue values based on half of the limit of detection for samples where nothing was detected.

Depending on the number of applications or work task of interest, the number of samples may be reduced by combining both upper limbs, both lower limbs and the chest/torso and back/torso. It is important to remember that the trouser tops (sectioned at upper thigh groin level) represent the lower part of the torso and therefore should be included with the upper garment.

**Variant of Whole Body Dosimeter Method for Use with Concurrent Biological Monitoring.** This variant of the whole body method involves the utilization of clothing as dosimeters to represent as closely as possible the normal work clothing of the worker population under study. Such clothing would include both the outer clothing (e.g. shirt and pants) and inner clothing (e.g. T-shirt and briefs). The method has particular merit in studies involving concurrent biological monitoring of the absorbed dose. Use of representative clothing ensures that there is no undue interference with the process of clothing penetration, dermal contamination and percutaneous absorption. The method and procedures used for sectioning and processing samples are essentially the same as those described for the standard whole body method. The key differences are in the calculations to estimate the dermal exposure.

## Hand Exposure

**Hand Rinse Method.** The selected solvent (previously evaluated for analytical suitability and human safety) should be placed in a polyethylene bag that is capable of withstanding vigorous shaking. The amount of solvent should be adequate to sample the entire hand. (The pesticide should be assessed for analytical compatibility with polyethylene before the field study.) A possible variation is to use a larger bag and wash both hands at the same time.

The bag should be held tightly at the wrist(s) of the subject and the hand(s) shaken vigorously approximately 50 times. Each hand should be rinsed a second time with fresh solvent and a new bag. Each bag and its solvent should then be placed in an individual appropriate container (e.g. mason jar or stainless steel container).

The hands of the worker should first be rinsed with the selected solvent prior to the field study, to remove any background contaminants.

During the course of the exposure study, hand rinses should be done each time the worker would normally wash his/her hands, as well as at the end of the day. Even if gloves are recommended on the product label, the worker should rinse his/her hands to establish whether any contamination occurred beneath the gloves.

If gloves are worn during the exposure study for a new product and it is not known whether gloves will be required on the label, it is recommended that both protective glove rinses and hand rinses be done. Rinses of the outside of the protective gloves should be done in the same manner as hand rinses, or full analysis of the protective gloves should be done in order to estimate potential hand exposure for workers not wearing gloves.

Any significant deviations from the standardized method described above should be adequately validated.

**Hand Wash with Soap and Water.** The hand wash method is recommended when exposure measurements and biological monitoring are to be conducted concurrently.

The subject should be asked to wash his/her hands as normal in 750 mL of water using a standardized soap in a clean plastic or stainless steel washing bowl.

The hands should then be rinsed with 250 mL of water. This is best achieved with assistance from a study investigator.

The soap and the procedure should have been validated in the laboratory for appropriate analytical recovery/extractability criteria.

The bowl may be reused for subsequent hand washes for the same subject, but not for other subjects.

Duplicate 200- or 250-mL aliquots of the pooled 1-L wash and rinse solutions should be taken and placed in suitable containers (e.g. glass or polyethylene) prior to frozen or cold storage. The containers should have been validated analytically in the laboratory for compatibility with the test material and the soap and water matrix.

The hand wash should be done whenever the worker normally washes his/her hands (e.g. before breaks and at the end of the working day). This ensures that there is no undue interference with the process of dermal hand contamination and percutaneous absorption.

**Absorbent Glove Method.** Lightweight absorbent gloves made of materials such as cotton should be selected for the study. To remove any substances that might interfere with pesticide residue analysis, gloves should be pre-tested and pre-extracted, if necessary, with the selected sample extraction solvent and allowed to dry before use. The practice of monitoring hand exposure by cutting sections from the palm or back of the absorbent gloves is not recommended, as hand exposure is often significant and the error in extrapolating from a smaller area to the whole hand may be large.

The hands of the worker should be washed thoroughly with soap and water or rinsed with a suitable solvent (e.g. distilled water, ethanol) to remove any interfering substances before he/she puts on the absorbent gloves.

If protective gloves are worn, the absorbent gloves should be worn beneath them.

If the absorbent gloves appear close to, or are anticipated to reach, saturation, they should be collected for analysis and a new pair of gloves used for the remainder of the day.

Absorbent gloves should be peeled off and replaced at times when the worker normally washes his/her hands and at the end of the work day and placed in an appropriate container (e.g. glass bottle, plastic bag).

Backup hand rinses, as described above in "Hand Rinse Method," may be required when hands are normally washed and at the end of the work day to sample pesticide residues that may have penetrated through the glove dosimeters, if the level of hand contamination or degree of saturation is suspected to be high.

It should be recognized that it is difficult to interpret the data from several sets of saturated absorbent gloves, because they have more absorption and retention capacity than the skin of the hands.

### Storage of Samples

All exposure samples should be stored temporarily in cool boxes containing dry ice or ice packs as necessary. They should be transferred to a deep-freeze as soon as possible. The times of sample collection and deposition in the deep-freeze should be recorded, as should all other essential sampling and storage information, and included in the Study File.

### Data Reporting and Calculations

All data (uncorrected and corrected where necessary for field recovery) should be reported in tables.

For each replicate, data should be presented in appropriate metric units such as mg or μg per patch or per body region (whole body dosimeter). Data for both inside and outside dosimeters should be reported.

In general, for values below the limit of detection of the analytical technique, one-half the limit of detection should be reported and used in the calculations.

Outside patch or uncovered whole body dosimeter data should be used for all uncovered body regions, whereas inside patch or whole body dosimeter data should be used for the body regions covered by normal work clothing and protective equipment.

**Calculations - Patch Method.** The μg/patch or mg/patch value should be divided by the exposed patch surface area ($cm^2$) to give the patch value in $\mu g/cm^2$ or $mg/cm^2$.

The $\mu g/cm^2$ or $mg/cm^2$ value should be multiplied by the corresponding regional body areas (Table A-1) to arrive at μg/body region or mg/body region.

Total potential dermal exposure should be calculated by summing the data based on the outer patches; estimated actual exposure should be calculated by summing the data from the inner patches.

**Calculations - Whole Body Methods.** Total potential dermal exposure should be calculated by summing the data for the individual outer and inner dosimeters.

Estimated actual exposure should be calculated in the following ways, depending on whether the normal work clothing of the worker population consists of one or two layers:

1. Where one layer of normal work clothing is worn, the data from the inner dosimeters can be summed to estimate exposure on the basis that they represent the skin.
2. Where two layers of clothing are worn over an inner dosimeter, dermal exposure is calculated as in 1., above.
3. Where two layers of clothing are worn, the residues on the outer and inner dosimeters can be used to estimate penetration through the inner sampling garment to the skin: i.e.

$$\text{Penetration factor (PF)} = \frac{\text{residue on inner dosimeter}}{\text{residues on outer + inner dosimeters}} \times 100$$

PFs for individual body parts can be used separately if the variance is large. Alternatively, a mean PF can be calculated from all the individual body parts per subject or even groups of subjects if the variance is small.

In studies involving concurrent biological monitoring, estimates of actual dermal exposure should include the dose estimated to have been absorbed percutaneously. In studies of use patterns where the dermal route of exposure is known to predominate, it can be assumed that all of the absorbed dose is derived from percutaneous absorption. The matter is more complicated for use patterns where the inhalation and/or oral routes are significant or if the pesticide is volatile. If inhalation exposure is measured, the percutaneously absorbed fraction can often be estimated by subtracting the inhaled dose from the total absorbed dose.

## INHALATION EXPOSURE

### Personal Air Sampling Method

It may be advisable to use a two-stage sampler if both vapours and aerosols are expected to be present. This should be determined during the sample medium selection process prior to the study, taking account of the physico-chemical properties of the pesticide. The vapour sampling medium would be located behind the aerosol sampling medium to collect any vapour stripped off the particulate during the sampling period.

The pump should be calibrated with the sampling device and collection medium in-line before and after each sampling period, and the flow rates should be reported for each replicate. Selection of a flow rate should reflect expected study conditions, considering such things as the length of the sampling replicate, concentration of pesticide in the air and retention of analyte. Typically, flow rates of 1-4 L/min are selected. For collection of the inspirable particulate using, for example, the IOM sampler, a flow rate of 2 L/min is a specific requirement.

The pump may be attached to the worker's belt. The sampling tube should be clipped on the lapel in the breathing zone of the worker. The placement of the tubing should not restrict the normal activities of the worker. The location of the sampling tube — i.e. left or right lapel — should be noted. It is advisable to standardize the location of the sampling tube or adjust its location according to whether the worker is left- or right-handed. The sampling tube should be pointed downward to simulate the anatomy of the nose and to prevent the collection of large droplets that would not normally be inhaled by the worker.

Unless potential for exposure continues during break and lunch periods, the sampling pump should be shut off during these times to provide a realistic measure of airborne concentrations of pesticide during the work periods.

The collection medium should be removed from the sampling tube at the end of the work day using suitable standardized methods that will not result in contamination.

### Storage of Samples

On completion of sampling, filter cassettes and tubes should be stored temporarily in a cool box containing dry ice or ice packs as necessary. The samples should be transferred to the deep-freeze as soon as possible after collection.

Inhalation exposure samples should be stored in cool boxes and freezer compartments separate from those used for dermal exposure, hand wash and urine samples.

### Data Reporting and Calculations

All data should be reported in tables.

All data, if necessary, should be corrected for field recovery.

For each replicate, data on the amount of pesticide found on the sampling medium should be presented in appropriate metric units, such as mg or μg per sampling tube or respirator.

For values below the limit of detection of the analytical technique, one-half the limit of detection should be reported.

Unless absorption information is available, 100% absorption is assumed for inhalation estimates.

The mean pump flow rate and exposure time for each replicate should be reported.

The airborne concentration should be calculated from:

$$\underset{(\mu g \text{ or } mg/L)}{\text{Concentration}} = \frac{\text{Amount found } (\mu g \text{ or } mg)}{\underset{(L/min)}{\text{Flow rate}} \times \underset{(min)}{\text{Sampling time}}} \times 1000 \text{ L}$$

The amount inhaled per replicate can be estimated by multiplying the airborne concentration by the appropriate ventilation rate for the work task. This can be obtained by reference to, for example, U.S. EPA's Exposure Factors Handbook (U.S. EPA, 1989). The selected ventilation rate should be adequately documented by the investigator.

## BIOLOGICAL MONITORING

### Urine Sampling

Urine sampling is the preferred method for biological monitoring in the field because it is non-invasive and because urine is relatively easy to collect.

Test subjects should be asked to ensure that they have no exposure to the test pesticide or structurally related product for an appropriate period of time before participating in the monitoring study. The appropriate period of time would be that required to ensure complete urinary clearance of the compound or any metabolites, based on the findings of the human volunteer dosing study. Ideally, subjects should handle no other pesticide during this period to circumvent the possibility of interference in the analyses of residues of the test material and/or its metabolites. It is recognized that this may not always be possible without undue interference with the working practices of the subjects; this, in turn, may affect their willingness to participate in the study.

Complete 24-hour urine collections should be obtained from subjects starting on the day before their use of the product, on the day(s) of use and for an appropriate period of time after use, depending upon the excretion kinetics of the compound. Urine samples should be collected in new, unused collection bottles specifically designed for this purpose. The material used in the construction of the collection bottles (e.g. polyethylene) should have been previously checked for analytical compatibility with the analytes of interest.

The 24-hour collection should start with the first void after commencing work activities on the day of use of the pesticide and finish with the first void the following morning. This cycle should be repeated for subsequent days' collections, with the first sample of the morning voided into the container issued the previous day. It is advisable to ensure that subjects understand that they must keep their containers available at all times throughout the day and collect all of their urine. Subjects should be told to exercise care in giving samples to avoid contamination of the urine with material present on their hands.

The total volume of each 24-hour sample should be measured, and two (e.g. 50 mL) aliquots should be taken and stored. One set of samples should be shipped to the laboratory for analysis while the other set remains in local deep-frozen storage as a reserve. All necessary precautions should be taken during sample collection and subsampling to avoid contamination of samples.

Specific issues that may arise and require consideration are (Woollen, 1993):

1. Volatility - if the pesticide or its metabolites are volatile, it may be necessary to take measures to minimize losses in the headspace in urine collection vessels.
2. Light sensitivity - if the pesticide or its metabolites are degraded by light, it may be necessary to use amber bottles.
3. Adsorption - polypropylene or polyethylene collection and storage vessels and caps are normally preferred, but glass bottles can be used if the pesticide or its metabolites bind or adsorb to polypropylene or polyethylene in the presence of urine. "Teflon" (or other inert) materials may be used for caps.
4. Temperature - the 24-hour stability of the compound and its metabolites at temperatures likely to be encountered in the field study must be known.
5. Preservatives - preservatives such as sodium azide are sometimes added to urine. Usually, samples can be frozen without preservatives.

## Blood Sampling

Blood monitoring to measure absorbed dose in workers occupationally exposed to pesticides has rarely been used because of the invasive nature of the collection method and the difficulty in obtaining a good correlation between blood concentrations and absorbed dose. The measurement of acetylcholinesterase (AChE) depression in plasma and red blood cells provides a semiquantitative measure of exposure to organophosphorus and carbamate pesticides. The usefulness of the measurement in quantitative risk assessment is limited unless a good correlation between level of AChE depression and systemic dose is demonstrated.

Where investigators believe that blood monitoring is warranted, the following specific blood collection and storage issues would need to be considered (Woollen, 1993):

1. Volatility - special procedures may be needed if the pesticide or its metabolites are volatile. A possible option is collection of blood in heparinized blood glass syringes, which can be sealed and centrifuged. Plasma could then be transferred to a vial for analysis using procedures that minimize losses into headspace.
2. Anticoagulants - possible interactions between the analytes and different anticoagulants should be considered. Lithium heparin is suitable for many applications.
3. Adsorption - adsorption of analytes to blood syringes or collection tubes should be investigated.
4. Centrifugation - a suitable centrifuge must be available at the site of the field study if plasma is required.
5. Infections - different containment requirements apply to handling blood samples from groups considered to be low, medium or high risk in relation to hepatitis B or HIV. If possible, potential donors should be screened for either or both of these infections before starting the study and excluded if positive. Otherwise, samples should be handled in accordance with the procedures recommended for medium- or high-risk blood samples according to local guidelines (e.g. ACDP, 1990). Particular attention should be given to packaging samples securely during transit; on receipt, samples should be opened in an appropriate containment facility.

## Data Reporting and Calculations

All data should be reported in tables. For each subject, the following data are required:

body weight in kg;
urine volume in mL and collection times;
urine volume in mL/24 h;
creatinine values in g/24 h.

A typical calculation of estimated absorption of a pesticide is as follows:

$$\text{estimated absorbed dose (mg)} = A\ (\text{mg}) \times \frac{M1}{M2} \times \frac{100}{R}$$

where:

A = total amount of metabolite in all urine samples collected;
M1 = molecular weight of pesticide;
M2 = molecular weight of metabolite;
R = average percent recovery of the administered dose excreted as metabolite in urine in human volunteer study.

A further correction would be needed if the metabolite degraded in stored urine or if urine collection was incomplete (i.e. to correct for compound and/or metabolites not yet excreted).

## SHIPMENT OF SAMPLES

Following completion of the field phase of the study, all samples should be shipped, if necessary in a deep-frozen or cold condition, to the laboratory for analysis. Because the samples must remain deep-frozen or cold, it is essential that proper, documented procedures be put into place to minimize the possibility of the samples thawing out or being lost in transit. The method and route of transit must therefore be known and arranged before shipment takes place. Appropriate "chain of custody" documentation should be used to satisfy GLP needs in these respects.

## TOTAL EXPOSURE AND ABSORBED DOSE CALCULATIONS AND INTERPRETATION

When the results have been compiled and tabulated, total potential and/or actual exposure should be calculated for each replicate. Field recovery results less than 95% should be used to correct the ambient exposure monitoring results. Recovery results greater than 95-100% should be noted but not used to correct the data.

### Passive Dosimetry

For calculating total exposure, all values for dermal deposition for each body region (including hands) should be summed for each replicate. The inhalation value should be treated separately. The sum is normalized by dividing by kg active ingredient (ai) handled. Each subject's exposure is expressed in terms of the appropriate standardized body weight (e.g. 70 kg).

Depending on the use conditions, exposure values may be normalized for other parameters, such as hectares (ha) treated, amount of produce treated (e.g. seed or wood) or time (h or min). This normalization is done to account for differences in work practices between individuals and for the variation in individual work practices during a full work day. It also standardizes all measured exposures to a common parameter, so that results can be compared between individuals.

The mean, range, standard deviation and coefficient of variation interval are calculated from the normalized results. Geometric mean, range and standard deviation may be calculated if the data are shown to be log-normally distributed. Other measures of central tendency may also be examined at the discretion of the investigator.

### Biological Monitoring

Normalization of biological monitoring absorbed dose data in terms of the parameters mentioned above under "Passive Dosimetry" might not be as appropriate as for ambient exposure data. This is because the assumption of direct proportionality between percutaneous, oral and inhalation absorptions and the standard parameters mentioned above may not be tenable. However, with this limitation in mind, the investigator may wish to examine the relationships between absorbed dose and these parameters.

Each subject's absorbed dose should be expressed in terms of body weight using his/her own measured value.

The arithmetic mean, range, standard deviation and coefficient of variation are calculated from the results. Geometric mean, range and standard deviation may be calculated if the results are shown to be log-normally distributed. Other measures of central tendency may also be examined at the discretion of the investigator.

## STUDY RECORDS

Standard forms may be used to document all parts of the field study, to cover the following aspects:

1. Personal details of subjects, including relevant agricultural experience;
2. Observations on work practice;
3. Trial location details, including site/field history and maps;
4. Details on number, size and design of formulation packs;
5. Details of application equipment;
6. Calibration of air sampling pumps;
7. Spray tank sampling;
8. Records of urine volumes and dates of collection and subsampling;
9. Study data form, including loading, weather and sampling information;
10. Field fortification of dermal and inhalation exposure sampling matrices;
11. Field fortification of urinary metabolite(s);
12. Deep-freeze sample deposition;
13. "Chain of custody" and other shipping information;
14. Incidents;
15. Study team personnel.

All the above documentation should be included in the Study File. Following completion of the field study, all study records should be indexed and, following preparation of the final report, transferred to a GLP Archive and stored for an indefinite period.

## REPORTING REQUIREMENTS

The following information is required:

1. Test material, purity, stability, product specification of formulation, batch numbers, nominal and actual concentrations;
2. Description of study design;
3. Exact locations of study sites, including site maps;
4. Description of mixing, loading and application equipment, application rate(s), crop areas treated/harvested;
5. Description of work procedures of workers, to include any use of protective clothing and equipment;
6. Detailed description of all sampling methods used, e.g. dermal, inhalation, biological monitoring, environmental conditions, field recovery evaluation;
7. Conditions of sample storage and shipment;
8. Description of analytical methodology, extraction, detection, validation;
9. Calculations and extrapolation factors;
10. Results of analysis, to include uncorrected and corrected residues, laboratory and field recoveries, extrapolated exposure and absorbed dose values, environmental conditions;
11. Tabulation of:
    All relevant analytical data;
    Extrapolation results, e.g. dermal, inhalation, exposure, absorbed dose (from biological monitoring);
    Environmental conditions;

12. Photographic record;
13. Discussion and interpretation of results;
14. Conclusions;
15. Location of raw data;
16. References.

## ANNEX II

## QUALITY ASSURANCE/QUALITY CONTROL

Quality Assurance/Quality Control data are required to support field studies of occupational exposure. These data fall into three areas:

1) "Pre-field Laboratory Considerations" covers those experiments associated with developing an analytical method for the analyte(s) of interest and validating its expected accuracy, precision and specificity in a specific sample matrix. This area includes determining the laboratory recovery efficiency, limit of detection and quantification and the working concentration range of the method. Recommended additional experiments include those determining the stability of the samples under the expected conditions of storage as well as the recovery from fortified samples exposed under simulated field conditions.

2) "Field Study Considerations" covers the major aspects of proper sample collection and validation. Sample collection needs include, but are not limited to, calibrating sampling equipment and ensuring that samples are properly handled and stored. Sample validation experiments include the preparation and collection of field recovery samples.

3) "Post-field Analytical Considerations" covers the need for regular laboratory instrument maintenance and calibration programs, the use of standard calibration curves to correct for day to day instrument variability, and the preparation and analysis of concurrent laboratory recovery samples to verify that the losses during extraction, clean-up, analysis, etc. are within acceptable limits as defined by the pre-field method validation work.

## PRE-FIELD LABORATORY CONSIDERATIONS

Analytical methods and sample collection procedures should be developed and validated before the field monitoring portion of a study is undertaken. Many aspects of the overall study design, such as the nature of the active ingredient and the end-use product in question, the proposed sampling technique(s) and duration, the anticipated time and conditions of sample storage, etc., can influence the method development and validation process. In addition, the relevant toxicological endpoints (acute and chronic) for the compound in question should be considered during the method development and validation phase of the study so that acceptable margins of safety can be demonstrated in the event that exposure samples yield values below the limit of detection or of quantification (LOD/LOQ).

## Analytical Method Validation

Analytical method validation establishes the performance of a particular method (e.g. the expected accuracy, precision, and specificity of a procedure for specific concentration ranges) within an analytical environment (e.g. within the laboratory that will perform the analysis of field samples). Method validation includes the analysis of a range of recovery samples for each matrix fortified with the neat analyte. Performance criteria should include a demonstration of the capability to attain reproducible results when measuring analytes at the desired level of sensitivity for all substrates prior to the initiation of field studies.

Minimally, the analytical method validation should include the following:

1. Establishment of the method's working concentration range to cover expected values from the field studies.
2. Determination of detector response over a reasonable standard concentration range.
3. Determination of the accuracy and precision of the method within the analytical environment through an experiment which should include the analysis of at least 7 replicates of each fortification level indicated below for each substrate.
    -- the method limit of quantitation (LOQ),
    -- an intermediate concentration level (e.g. 10X LOQ),
    -- the maximum concentration of the validation range (e.g. 100 - 1000X LOQ), and
    -- blank or control substrate.

An accuracy value between 70-120 percent (average recovery) and a precision value less than or equal to 20 percent (coefficient of variation) demonstrates the analytical laboratory's capability to perform accurate and precise analysis.

The necessary LOQ will depend on the toxicological endpoint of interest. At a very minimum the LOQ should be sufficient to assess exposures at the no-observed-effect level (NOEL) divided by an appropriate safety factor. It is desirable and recommended that the LOQ be sufficient to quantify exposures well below the NOEL divided by an appropriate safety factor.

## Post Method Validation Studies

**Storage Stability.** A storage stability study can be conducted prior to or in conjunction with a field study. Its purpose is to determine the stability of analyte(s) in or on appropriate sample matrices under similar storage conditions that will be used to store field samples. Conducting a storage stability study prior to study initiation may eliminate the need for generating storage recovery data during the field study.

A storage stability study should include the following parameters:

- preparation and analysis of at least 3 blanks, 3 low-level fortifications (2-10X the LOQ), and 3 high level fortifications in the expected range of field samples for each storage interval, including the longest interval planned for storage of field samples; and
- storage of samples under the same conditions of storage as planned for the field samples (e.g., sample matrices or extracts, ambient temperature and/or frozen).

A storage stability study, done before, or in conjunction with the field study, is optional if the field recovery samples are stored and analyzed with the actual field samples.

**Pre-Trial Field Recovery.** A pre-trial field recovery study is recommended in some cases. The purpose of a pre-trial field recovery study is to estimate the potential loss of analyte from sample collection devices, when subjected to environmental conditions (e.g. temperature, light, relative humidity, wind) and sample durations representative of those anticipated during collection of the actual field exposure samples. This study may be done under actual or simulated field conditions. Laboratory incubators can be used to simulate anticipated field temperature and humidity conditions. If environmental conditions are anticipated to change during the actual field study, then a worst-case scenario (i.e. most chances for volatilization/degradation) should be used.

### Sample Collection Devices

During pre-field study design, investigators should give consideration to selecting the most appropriate sample collection devices and methodologies available for monitoring the pesticides and use scenarios in question. The following should be considered:

- dermal dosimeters and other sample collection devices should be durable enough to survive the physical stress and duration of the overall monitoring procedure, including sample collection, transportation and analysis. In addition, reasonable judgement should be used in the selection of sample collection devices to ensure that their absorptive capacity is not exceeded (i.e. become saturated) during the sample collection process.
- sampling media should be selected that do not contain substances that might interfere with analysis. Pre-extraction may be required to remove coextractants and contaminating substances.

## FIELD CONSIDERATIONS

Field recovery samples are collected, handled, transported and stored in conjunction with the experimental samples and account for losses that occur during all phases of sample collection, sample handling and storage in the field, transportation from the field to the laboratory and storage in the laboratory. Additionally, field recovery samples that are analyzed concurrently with the experimental samples account for residue losses that occur during sample extraction and analysis. Travel recovery samples can also be prepared in the field and shipped and stored with the experimental samples. The results of the travel recovery samples provide a basis for estimating the losses that occur during sample shipment and storage as opposed to those which occur during sample collection. The inclusion of travel recovery samples is recommended, but not essential.

### Field Recovery of Exposure Samples

Field recovery refers to data generated to determine the loss of analyte from sample collection devices fortified in the field, when subjected to the same environmental conditions (e.g. temperature, light, relative humidity, wind) and duration as field exposure samples.

Ideally, a separate set of field recovery samples should be collected at each site on each day of monitoring. However, it may be acceptable to collect a single set of field recovery samples for all replicates monitored on the same day at different sites provided that ambient conditions are similar. It may also be acceptable to collect a single set of field recovery samples for all replicates monitored at a given site over the course of a few days if the environmental conditions are similar each day. This approach is recommended for compounds that are very stable only, and in locations where the climate does not change appreciably from one day to the next during monitoring. The investigator who chooses this approach to generating field recovery data should demonstrate the stability of the compound as well as the day-to-day consistency of the climate at the study site(s).

A complete set of field recoveries should consist of 3 or more each of blank control samples, low level fortifications, and high level fortifications. More than 3 samples may be warranted for compounds known to be unstable in the field or having little history of field evaluation. The low and high level fortifications should be in the range of the anticipated level of the chemical on the substrate. If the highest expected level is more than 100X the lowest spiking level, it is recommended that a mid-level of fortification be included.

It is advisable to generate sufficient field recovery samples to be analyzed at the same time as the actual field samples to serve as concurrent laboratory recovery samples. At a minimum, a complete set of field recoveries, preferably fortified with the formulated product would consist of the following, when applicable:

1. Air sampling matrices. The analyte should be added to the collection matrices in the field at the time of the study. After fortification and evaporation of the delivery solvent, the fortified matrices should be exposed to ambient conditions and attached to air pumps. The pumps should be operated in clean air at a flow rate, and for the length of time, equivalent to the field samples.
2. Patches. The number of patches is irrespective of whether the worker wears one patch or 22 patches. However, if some of the patches are covered by clothing (inside patches versus outside patches), a separate set of fortified patches may be prepared and covered by clothing during the exposure period at the control site.
3. Whole Body Dosimeters (WBDs). Pieces of test garments should be used for fortification as field recovery samples and controls. Investigators should use discretion when preparing samples. For example, investigators could split a garment designated for QC purposes into samples that are reflective of the field samples (e.g. arms or legs) or into smaller fabric swatches (e.g. 100 $cm^2$) and fortify the individual samples. Exposed WBDs, such as coveralls are to be fortified at both the low level and the high level. Covered items may only need to be fortified at the low level, covered, and exposed to the elements at the control site.

   However, several issues exist which should be considered:

   - fortification levels must reflect the relative size of the QC fabric swatch samples compared to a typical field sample (i.e. the fortification level should be similar to the anticipated field sample levels on a per area basis as analytical background may be important in the data interpretation).
   - the total solvent extraction volume should be proportional to the surface area for both the field exposure samples and the field recovery samples (e.g. if a solvent volume of 1,000 mL is used to

extract a 2,000 $cm^2$ section of a field exposure sample then a solvent volume of 50 mL should be used to extract a 100 $cm^2$ field recovery swatch).

- QC sample swatches must be generated from the same production lots of dosimeters and prepared in the same manner (e.g. pre-extraction) as the monitors used to collect the actual field samples.
- the quantitation limit for each particular matrix must be considered when specifying fortification levels (e.g. the determination of low fortification levels when prorating based on the surface area of the sample). The use of the fabric swatches will conserve considerable storage space and solvent usage. The similarity of recoveries should be established during method development and validation. If it is established that the fortification of fabric swatches yields results similar to whole sections of the WBD, it is acceptable to use swatches for field recovery samples.

4. Gloves, socks, briefs, head bands, etc. Exposed clothing items, such as gloves (if used as a dosimeter), should be fortified at both the low level and the high level. Covered items, such as briefs, may only need to be fortified at the low level, covered, and exposed to the elements at the control site.
5. Hand rinses. It is not appropriate to expose hand rinse samples to the environment during the field phase of a study since they are collected, processed, and stored immediately, without significant exposure to the elements. However, all samples should be handled using the same procedures as the actual field samples. For example, fortified hand rinse solutions should be "set out," for as long as it takes to conduct a hand wash, prior to storage or packing for shipment.
6. Urine/Blood. If urine or blood is collected for biological monitoring, it is recommended that at least 3 samples of control (non-participant or pre-participation) urine or blood be fortified at each of 2 levels of the analyte (parent or metabolite(s), whichever is appropriate) for each experimental site. These fortifications may be made just prior to going to the field, carried into the field, exposed in a manner similar to participants' urine or blood, and stored and shipped with experimental samples. If stability of the analyte(s) has been rigorously established prior to study initiation, investigators may choose to reduce or eliminate this component from the study design because it is a burdensome task.

**Travel Recovery**

Travel recovery samples refer to data from experiments conducted to determine the stability of the analyte on each sampling matrix during shipment and possibly storage. Travel recovery samples are optional and are left up to the discretion of the investigator. These recovery samples are prepared concurrently with the field portion of the study. They are then shipped and stored with the appropriate experimental samples. The travel recovery samples are different than field recovery samples in that they are not exposed to the environmental conditions during the sample collection period. Thus, the results of the travel recovery samples reflect losses which may occur during shipment and storage only as opposed to those which occur during sample collection, shipment and storage. It is suggested that one set of travel recovery samples be prepared for each experimental site to aid in the interpretation of losses that may occur in field recovery samples. If field recovery samples indicate no significant losses, the travel recovery samples do not need to be analyzed.

### Fortification of Sampling Matrices

If the pesticide is to be applied as a spray, the fortification of exposure sampling devices should be made with the formulated pesticide product diluted in the spray matrix (usually water). For products applied as a solid (granules, pellets), or for formulations in which it is difficult to get a uniform suspension, and for air sampling media, it is recommended that a solution of the analyte usually in an organic solvent, be used. Such a solution is also recommended for fortifying hand rinse solutions and for fortifying urine samples (analyte or metabolite).

### Spray Tank Sample Analysis

During the study, an appropriate number of tank mix samples should be taken and analyzed to verify the application rate, and the amount of active ingredient loaded and applied per tank.

### Quality Control and Sample Generation

Any sample collection equipment used in a study by an investigator should be validated and/or calibrated. Examples include: personal sampling pumps should be calibrated using a device which is traceable to a primary standard (e.g. bubble meter or, magnahelic or "Buck" type Calibrator); thermometers used in any study must be traceable to a NIST primary standard; and weights used to calibrate analytical balances should be traceable to NIST primary standards (e.g. class P or better).

## POST-FIELD ANALYTICAL CONSIDERATIONS

The basis for any modern analytical method is the instrumentation. Instrumental methods that are both sensitive and stable should be developed. Peaks of interest should readily be separated from contaminant peaks by intervals (e.g. time, wavelength, etc.) that are large enough to allow for accurate resolution and quantification of the peaks of interest. The lowest level analytical (i.e. calibration) standard should produce a signal that is at least three times greater in magnitude than the signal to noise ratio. In other words, the instrumental signal to noise ratio must be $\geq 3$ for the lowest standard.

### Instrument Performance

Instrument performance must be monitored regularly to ensure the reliability of the measurements. Several techniques that can be used to establish instrument performance include, but are not limited to: (1) internal standards, (2) daily comparison of peak areas of analytical standards, or (3) calculation of a correlation coefficient for a particular standard curve. Investigators must establish their own guidelines for determining whether an instrument is functioning properly, as this determination is dependent upon the analytical method, instrument operating parameters, and background levels observed/anticipated in the samples.

Determining the proper instrument operational quality control procedures is difficult. Investigators must develop operational standards that are pertinent to the pesticide(s) being studied (e.g. detector response patterns affect calibration techniques).

Investigators must also develop criteria for scrutinizing daily method performance data. It is recognized that recovery results are proportional to the extraction and instrumental methods as well as the physical/chemical characteristics of the pesticide(s) being studied. Therefore, studies for which the recovery results are marginal should be considered on a case-by-case basis. Investigators should be careful to provide justifications as to why their analytical methods and results appear to be marginal.

### Calibration Techniques

As described above, results can be calculated in a variety of ways. Interpretation of basic results, however, demands generating a standard (i.e. calibration) curve to which responses from sample extracts can be compared. If calculations are to be done manually, for example, a linear regression analysis can be performed. Investigators should describe all techniques used to calibrate instruments and calculate residue levels. Data integration systems, besides enabling investigators to manipulate/interpret data in a variety of ways (i.e. various peak integration techniques), also typically generate calibration curves as well as calculate and summarize results. Several options for generating calibration curves are usually available in each system (e.g. linear regression for all points, point to point calibration, average values based on multiple analysis, etc.). Investigators must be careful to consider the response patterns of a particular instrumental system (i.e. linear, exponential, threshold, etc.) prior to selecting a means to generate the calibration curve.

### Concurrent Laboratory Recovery

Concurrent laboratory recovery data are data analyzed in the analytical laboratory at the same time as the field samples to determine the recovery efficiency of the analyte from substrates and the day to day variation in the method sensitivity. Laboratory recoveries, typically fortified with analytical standards reflect losses which occur during laboratory operations (extraction, clean-up, analytical measurement, etc.). They do not account for losses which occur during sample collection, shipping or storage. It is recommended that a minimum of 10 percent of the field samples be represented by a laboratory recovery sample for each analytical batch/run, and they should cover the range of concentrations anticipated in field samples.

Concurrent laboratory recovery samples can be either field recovery samples analyzed concurrently with the actual field samples or laboratory samples generated (i.e. fortified) in the laboratory. It is recommended that the field recovery samples be used as concurrent laboratory samples. When used in this manner, the field recovery samples could be used to correct the field samples for both losses in the field and laboratory. However, if the investigator is not confident of the fate of the compound in the field and during storage, recovery samples generated in the laboratory should be used to identify where the losses may have occurred (i.e. field or analytical method).

## ANNEX III

## GLOSSARY OF TERMS

**active ingredient:**

That ingredient of a pesticide to which the pest control effects of the pesticide are primarily attributed.

**actual dermal exposure:**

The amount of pesticide coming into contact with bare (uncovered) skin and the fraction transferring through protective and work clothing or via seams to the underlying skin, and which is therefore available for percutaneous absorption.

**ambient monitoring:**

A method of measuring the amount of a substance that is available for uptake: composed of environmental monitoring and personal monitoring.

**analyte:**

Chemical moiety (pesticide or metabolite) that is the subject of chemical analysis.

**applicator:**

A person actively engaged in the application of the pesticide.

**arithmetic mean:**

A value that is computed by dividing the sum of a set of terms by the number of terms, i.e. $\frac{X_1 + X_2 + ... + X_n}{n}$.

**biological monitoring:**

A method of assessing the absorption of chemicals by measuring the parent compound or its metabolites in body fluids, usually blood, urine or exhaled breath.

Woollen (1993) refined this term in the context of pesticides and assessment of absorbed dose for risk assessment: "Measurement of a pesticide or its metabolites in the body fluids of exposed persons and conversion to an equivalent absorbed dose of the pesticide based on a knowledge of its human metabolism and pharmacokinetics."

**breakthrough:**

The passage of a chemical through a sampling medium (e.g. air sampling tube) or penetration of a chemical through protective clothing or devices (e.g. gloves, respirator).

**breathing zone:**

The area around the nose and mouth from which air is inhaled.

**bystander:**

A person potentially exposed to pesticides but not necessarily engaged in the application procedure.

**closed system:**

A system of mixing and/or loading and transfer in which the chemical is isolated from the ambient environment at all points from the original container to the spray tank.

**cycle:**

A recurring sequence composed of one mixing, one loading and one application event.

**dermal absorption:**

Movement of a pesticide into and through the skin; includes that taken up into the systemic circulation and that retained in the skin compartment.

**dislodgeable residue:**

Residue of an applied pesticide that may be removed from a treated or untreated surface by solvent rinse.

**dose:**

The amount of a pesticide systemically available.

**drift:**

The movement of pesticide by wind or air currents to non-target areas.

**environmental monitoring:**

A method of measuring the amount of a pesticide present in an environmental medium.

**exposure:**
A condition of oral, dermal, respiratory or ocular contact between a person and a pesticide.

**extrapolation:**
Quantitative estimate of values outside the range of measured values.

**field blank:**
A sampling device subjected to the same conditions as the field samples but not exposed to the product under study.

**field recovery:**
The recovery of analyte from sample collection devices fortified and subjected to the same environmental conditions, exposure times, handling, shipping, storage and laboratory operations as field exposure samples.

**flagger:**
A person engaged in marking the border between treated and untreated areas during pesticide application.

**formulation:**
A mixture of an active ingredient with diluents, carriers and other materials to form the packaged product.

**geometric mean:**
The nth root of the product of n numbers, i.e. $(X_1 \times X_2 \ldots X_n)^{1/n}$.

**inspirable fraction:**
That fraction of airborne particulate capable of entering the respiratory tract via the nose and the mouth, so providing a source of absorption into the body, either from direct inhalation or from subsequent oral ingestion.

**label:**
Any legend, word, mark, symbol or design applied or attached to, included in, belonging to or accompanying any control product.

**laboratory recovery:**
The recovery of the analyte from sample collection devices fortified in the laboratory; refers to laboratory operations only and does not refer to losses due to storage conditions or environmental factors.

**limit of detection:**
The level at which a pesticide can be detected but not quantified for a given analytical procedure.

**limit of quantification:**
The smallest amount of the pesticide that can be quantified by the analytical method.

**mixer-loader:**
A person who mixes and/or loads but does not necessarily apply a pesticide.

**normalization:**
A standardized expression of exposure as a function of another variable (e.g. μg/amount active ingredient handled, μg/time, μg/area treated).

**passive dosimetry:**
A method of measuring the amount of pesticide coming into contact with an individual.

**personal monitoring:**
(see passive dosimetry)

**pesticide:**
Any substance or mixture of substances intended for preventing or controlling any unwanted species of plants and animals; also includes any substances or mixture of substances intended for use as a plant growth regulator, defoliant or desiccant.

**pharmacokinetics:**
The study of the absorption, distribution, metabolism and excretion of a substance in any living system.

**potential dermal exposure:**
The total amount of pesticide coming into contact with the protective clothing, work clothing and skin.

**reentry period:**
A period of time that elapses before an individual reenters a treated area, or the period of time that defines when individuals may reenter a treated area.

**replicate:**
A measurement of exposure to a worker during one typical work day, which includes all job functions related to pesticide use.

**site:**
A location at which one or more replicates are monitored.

**storage stability:**
The recovery of analyte from sample collection devices fortified and subjected to the same handling, shipping, storage and laboratory operations as field exposure samples.

**surrogate data:**
Exposure data collected for one pesticide that are used to estimate exposure to a similar pesticide.

**ventilation rate:**
Breathing rate used for calculating inhalation exposure.

**worker:**
Person engaged in work activities associated with possible exposure to pesticides.

## ANNEX IV

## REVISION COMMITTEE

| | | |
|---|---|---|
| Graham Chester | - | Zeneca Agrochemicals, United Kingdom |
| Patricia Curry | - | Health Canada, Canada |
| John Worgan | - | Health Canada, Canada |
| Pamela Maloney | - | Health Canada, Canada |

## PEER REVIEW COMMITTEE

| | | |
|---|---|---|
| Neil Carmichael | - | Rhone Poulenc Agro Chimie, France |
| Monty Eberhart | - | Miles Inc., USA |
| Richard Fenske | - | University of Washington, USA |
| Curt Lunchick | - | Jelinek, Swartz and Connolly, USA |
| Wolfgang Maasfeld | - | Bayer AG, Germany |
| Marco Maroni | - | Internationale Centre for Pesticide Safety, Italy |
| Alan Nielsen | - | US Environmental Protection Agency, USA |
| John Ross | - | California Environmental Protection Agency, USA |
| Joop van Hemmen | - | TNO Nutrition and Food Research, The Netherlands |

## REFERENCES


Abbott, I.M., Bonsall, J.L., Chester, G., Hart, T.B., and Turnbull, G.J., 1987, Worker exposure to a herbicide applied with ground sprayers in the United Kingdom, *Am. Ind. Hyg. Assoc. J.* 48:167-175.

ACDP, Advisory Committee on Dangerous Pathogens, 1990, "Categorisation of Pathogens According to Hazard and Categories of Containment," HMSO, London.

Alessio, L., Bolin, A., Dell'Orto, A., Toffoletto, F., and Ghezzio, I., 1985, Reliability of urinary creatinine as a parameter used to adjust values of urinary biological indicators, *Int. Arch. Occup. Environ. Health* 55:99-106.

Berkow, S.G., 1931, Value of surface area proportions in the prognosis of cutaneous burns and scalds, *Am. J. Surg.* 11:315-317.

Boeniger, M.F., Lowry, L.K., and Rosenberg, J., 1993, Interpretation of urine results used to assess chemical exposure with emphasis on creatinine adjustments: A review, *Am. Ind. Hyg. Assoc. J.* 54(10):615-627.

Carmichael, N.G., 1995, Pesticide exposure: Overview of the tiered approach, *in*: "Proceedings of the Workshop on Methods of Pesticide Exposure Assessment," October 5-8, 1993, Ottawa, Canada.

Chester, G., 1993, Evaluation of agricultural worker exposure to, and absorption of, pesticides, *Ann. Occup. Hyg.* 37(5):509-523.

Chester, G., and Hart, T.B., 1986, Biological monitoring of a herbicide applied through backpack and vehicle sprayers, *Toxicol. Lett.* 33:137-149.

Chester, G., Dick, J., Loftus, N.J., Woollen, B.H., and Anema, B.H., 1990, The effectiveness of protective gloves in reducing dermal exposure to, and absorption of, the herbicide fluazifop-p-butyl by mixer-loader-applicators using tractor sprayers, *in*: "Proceedings of the 7th International Congress of Pesticide Chemistry," Vol. III, IUPAC.

Curry, P., and Iyengar, S., 1992, Comparison of exposure assessment guidelines for pesticides, *Rev. Environ. Contam. Toxicol.* 129:79-93.

Davis, J.E., 1980, Minimizing occupational exposure to pesticides: Personal monitoring, *Residue Rev.* 75:35-50.

Durham, W.F., and Wolfe, H.T., 1962, Measurement of the exposure of workers to pesticides, *Bull. WHO* 26:75-91.

Fenske, R.A., 1990, Non-uniform dermal deposition patterns during occupational exposure to pesticides, *Arch. Environ. Contam. Toxicol.* 19:332-337.

Fenske, R.A., 1993, Dermal exposure assessment techniques, *Ann. Occup. Hyg.* 37:687-706.

Fenske, R.A., and Lu, C., 1994, Determination of handwash removal efficiency; incomplete removal of the pesticide chlorpyrifos from skin by standard handwash techniques, *Am. Ind. Hyg. Assoc. J.* 55(5):425-432.

Fenske, R.A., Leffingwell, J.T., and Spear, R.C., 1986a, A video imaging technique for assessing dermal exposure - I. Instrument design and testing, *Am. Ind. Hyg. Assoc. J.* 47:764-770.

Fenske, R.A., Wong, S.M., Leffingwell, J.T., and Spear, R.C., 1986b, A video imaging technique for assessing dermal exposure - II. Fluorescent tracer testing, *Am. Ind. Hyg. Assoc. J.* 47:771-775.

Fenske, R.A., Birnbaum, S.G., and Cho, K., 1990, Documentation for a second generation video imaging technique for assessing dermal exposure, Rutgers University Department of Environmental Science, New Brunswick, N.J.

GIFAP, Groupement International des Associations Nationales de Fabricants de Produits Agrochimiques, 1990, "Monitoring Studies in the Assessment of Field Worker Exposure to Pesticides," Technical Monograph No. 14, Bruxelles, Belgium.

Grover, R., Franklin, C.A., Muir, N.I., Cessna, A.J., and Riedel, D., 1986, Dermal exposure and urinary metabolite excretion in farmers repeatedly exposed to 2,4-D amine, *Toxicol. Lett.* 33:73-83.

Henderson, P.Th., Brouwer, D.H., Opdam, J.J.G., Stevenson, H., and Stouten, J.Th.J., 1993, Risk assessment for worker exposure to agricultural pesticides: Review of a workshop, *Ann. Occup. Hyg.* 37(5):499-507.

Lewis, R.G., 1976, Sampling and analysis of airborne pesticides, *in*: "Air Pollution from Pesticides and Agricultural Processes," R.E. Lee, Jr., ed., CRC Press, Cleveland, Ohio.

Lundehn, J.-R., Westphal, D., Kieczka, H., Krebs, B., Löcher-Bolz, S., Massfeld, W., and Pick, E.-D., 1992, "Uniform Principles for Safeguarding the Health of Applicators of Plant Protection Products," Mitteilungen aus der Biologischen Bundesanstalt für Land-und Forstwirtschaft, Heft 277, Berlin, Germany.

Martin, A.D., 1990, A predictive model for the assessment of dermal exposure to pesticides, *in*: "Prediction of Percutaneous Penetration. Methods, Measurements, Modelling," R.C. Scott, R.H. Guy, and J. Hadgraft, eds., IBC Technical Services Ltd., Southampton.

Melcher, R.G., Garner, W.L., Severs, L.W., and Vaccaro, J.R., 1978, Collection of chlorpyrifos and other pesticides in air on chemically bonded sorbents, *Anal. Chem.* 50(2):215-225.

Mull, R., and McCarthy, J.F., 1986, Guidelines for conducting mixer- loader-applicator studies, *Vet. Hum. Toxicol.* 28(4):328-336.

NACA, National Agricultural Chemicals Association, 1985, "Guidelines for Conducting Biological Monitoring - Applicator Exposure Studies," NACA, Washington, D.C.

National Academy of Sciences, 1983, "Risk Assessment in the Federal Government: Managing the Process," National Academy Press, Washington, D.C.

OECD, Organisation for Economic Co-operation and Development, 1992, "GLP Consensus Document. The Application of the GLP Principles to Field Studies," Environment Monograph No. 50, OECD Series on Principles of Good Laboratory Practice and Compliance Monitoring No. 6.

Peoples, S.A., and Knaak, J., 1982, Monitoring pesticide blood cholinesterase and analysing blood and urine for pesticides and their metabolites, *in*: "Pesticide Residues and Exposure," J.R. Plimmer, ed., ACS Symp. Series No. 182, American Chemical Society, Washington, D.C.

PHED, 1992, Pesticide Handlers Exposure Database, U.S. Environmental Protection Agency, Health and Welfare Canada, National Agricultural Chemicals Association.

Ritter, L., and Franklin, C.A., 1989, Use of biological monitoring in the regulatory process, *in*: "Biological Monitoring for Pesticide Exposure," R.G.M. Wang, C.A. Franklin, R.C. Honeycutt, and J.C. Reinert, eds., ACS Symp. Series No. 382, American Chemical Society, Washington, D.C.

Thongsinthusak, T., Ross, J.H., and Meinders, D., 1993, "Guidance for the Preparation of Human Pesticide Exposure Documents," HS-1612, May 4, California Environmental Protection Agency, Worker Health and Safety Branch.

U.S. EPA, Environmental Protection Agency, 1985, "Pesticide Assessment Guidelines, Subdivision K. Exposure: Re-entry Protection," U.S. EPA, Washington, D.C.

U.S. EPA, Environmental Protection Agency, 1987, "Pesticide Assessment Guidelines, Subdivision U, Applicator Exposure Monitoring," U.S. EPA, Washington, D.C.

U.S. EPA, Environmental Protection Agency, 1989, "Exposure Factors Handbook," Office of Health and Environmental Assessment, EPA/600/08-89/043.

Van Dyk, L.P., and Visweswariah, K., 1975, Pesticides in air: Sampling methods, *Residue Rev.* 55:91-134.

Van Heemstra-Lequin, E.A.H., and Van Sittert, N.J., eds., 1986, "Biological Monitoring of Workers Manufacturing, Formulating and Applying Pesticides," *Toxicol. Lett.* 33, Elsevier, Amsterdam.

van Hemmen, J.J., 1992, Agricultural pesticide exposure databases for risk assessment, *Rev. Environ. Contam. Toxicol.* 126:1-85.

Vincent, J.H., and Mark, D., 1987, Comparison of criteria for defining inspirable aerosol and the development of appropriate samplers, *Am. Ind. Hyg. Assoc. J.* 48:451-457.

Wang, R.G.M., Franklin, C.A., Honeycutt, R.C., and Reinert, J.C., 1989, "Biological Monitoring for Pesticide Exposure: Measurement, Estimation and Risk Reduction," ACS Symp. Series No. 382, American Chemical Society, Washington, D.C.

Watts, P., and Chen, W., 1995, European Operator Exposure Database, *in*: "Proceedings of the Workshop on Methods of Pesticide Exposure Assessment," October 5-8, 1993, Ottawa, Canada.

WHO, World Health Organization, 1975, "Survey of Exposure to Organophosphorus Pesticides in Agriculture. Standard Protocol," VBC/75.9, WHO, Geneva.

WHO, World Health Organization, 1982, "Field Surveys of Exposure to Pesticides. Standard Protocol," VBC/82.1, WHO, Geneva.

Wolfe, H.R., 1976, Field exposure to airborne pesticides, *in*: "Air Pollution from Pesticides and Agricultural Processes," R.E. Lee, Jr., ed., CRC Press, Cleveland, Ohio.

Woollen, B.H., 1993, Biological monitoring for pesticide absorption, *Ann. Occup. Hyg.* 37(5):525-540.

## WORKSHOP PARTICIPANTS

Bystedt, Margareta
Swedish National Chemicals
Inspectorate
Solna, SWEDEN

Carmichael, Neil G.
Rhone Poulenc Secteur Agro
Sophia Antipolis Cedex
FRANCE

Chang, Fa-yan
Agriculture Canada
Ottawa, CANADA

Chester, Graham
Zeneca Agrochemicals
Surrey, UNITED KINGDOM

Chu, Ih
Health Canada
Ottawa, CANADA

Coates, B.
Crop Protection Institute
Etobicoke, CANADA

Curry, Patricia B.
Health Canada
Ottawa, CANADA

Day, Edgar W.
DowElanco
Indianapolis, USA

Delgado Cobos, Pedro
Inst. National de Seguridad e
Higiene en el Trabajo - CNMP
Sevilla, SPAIN 41080

Dorsey, Larry
US Environmental Protection Agency
Washington, USA

Eberhart, Delmont C.
Miles Inc.
Kansas City, USA

Fait, Antonella
International Centre for Pesticide
Safety
Busto Garolfo, ITALY

Fenske, Richard A.
University of Washington
Seattle, USA

Forget, Gilles
International Development Research
Corporation
Ottawa, CANADA

Foster, Kent
Health Canada
Ottawa, CANADA

Franklin, Claire
Health Canada
Vanier, CANADA

Gee, Shirley J.
University of California
Davis, USA

Grissom, Raymond E.
Agency for Toxic Substances &
Disease Registry
Atlanta, USA

Hamey, Paul
Pesticides Safety Directorate
York, UNITED KINGDOM

Hoernicke, Eberhard
Federal Biological Research
Centre
Kleinmachnew, GERMANY

Iyengar, Seshadri
Zeneca Agro
Stoney Creek, CANADA

Kashyap, Shri Kant
National Institute of
Occupational Health
Ahmedabad, INDIA

Koëter, Herman B.W.M.
Organisation for Economic
Cooperation and Development
Paris, FRANCE

Krebs, Berthold
Hoechst AG
Frankfurt/Main 80,
GERMANY

Krieger, Robert I.
University of California
Riverside, USA

Leighton, Tim
Versar Inc.
Springfield, USA

Leist, Karl Heinz
Hoechst Aktiengesellschaft
Hattersheim, GERMANY

Lunchick, Curt
Jellinek, Schwartz & Connolly
Arlington, USA

Maas, Chris
Ministry of Social Affairs &
Employment
Den Haag, THE NETHERLANDS

Maasfeld, Wolfgang
Bayer AG
Leverkusen, GERMANY

Maloney, Pamela
Health Canada
Ottawa, CANADA

Maroni, Marco
International Centre for Pesticide
Safety
Busto Garolfo, ITALY

Miri, Minoo
The University of Canterbury
Kent, UNITED KINGDOM

Moore, Gregory
National Chemcials Inspectorate
Solna, SWEDEN

Morison, Deirdre
Health Canada
Ottawa, CANADA

Mull, Ron
Du Pont AG Products
Wilmington, USA

Murray, Bill
Food & Agriculture Organization
of the United Nations
Rome, ITALY

Nielsen, Alan
US Environmental Protection Agency
Washington, USA

Nielsen, Kjeld Mann
Danish Working Environment
Service
Copenhagen, DENMARK

Pontal, Pierre-Gérard
Rhone Poulenc Agro Chimie
Lyon, FRANCE

Purdy, John
CIBA Canada
Mississauga, CANADA

Ritter, Leonard
Canadian Network of Toxicology
Centres
Guelph, CANADA

Robinson, Ann E.
WHO - International Program on
Chemical Safety
Toronto, CANADA

Ross, John H.
California Environmental Protection
Agency
Sacramento, USA

Schulze, Corina
CIBA-GEIGY Ltd.
Basle, SWITZERLAND

Seligy, Vern
Health Canada
Ottawa, CANADA

Smeets, Louis
Commission of the European
Communities
Bruxelles, BELGIUM

Smith, Megan
Worksafe Australia
Sydney, AUSTRALIA

Sorup Hansen, Nina
Danish EPA
Copenhagen, DENMARK

Straight, Michael
Allergy Respiratory Institute of
Colorado
Denver, USA

van Hemmen, Joop J.
TNO Nutrition and Food Research
Rijswijk, THE NETHERLANDS

Warfield, Chris
Health Canada
Ottawa, CANADA

Watts, Peter
BIBRA International
Surrey, UNITED KINGDOM

Westphal, Dieter
Bundesgesundheitsamt
Berlin, GERMANY

Woollen, Bruce
Zeneca Central Toxicology
Laboratory
Cheshire, UNITED KINGDOM

Worgan, John P.
Health Canada
Ottawa, CANADA

# INDEX

o-o-AC-199